Stay curious!

Cait Lynch

NOURISH
What Are You Hungry For?

by

Cait Lynch

Nourish
Copyright © 2016 Cait Lynch
All rights reserved
Published by Blue Denim Press Inc.
First Edition
ISBN 978-1-927882-16-0.

The ideas, procedures and suggestions contained in this book are not intended as a substitute for consulting your physician. All matters regarding your health require medical supervision.

The poem "Autobiography in Five Short Chapters" by Portia Nelson is reprinted here with the permission of Simon & Schuster, Inc.

Cover Design–Joanna Joseph/Typeset in Helvetica and Garamond
Library and Archives Canada Cataloguing in Publication

Lynch, Cait, author
    NOURISH : What Are You Hungry For? / Cait Lynch.

Includes bibliographical references.
Issued in print and electronic formats.
ISBN 978-1-927882-16-0 (paperback).--ISBN 978-1-927882-17-7 (epub).--ISBN 978-1-927882-18-4 (kindle)

    1. Health. 2. Health behavior. 3. Self-care, Health. I. Title.

RA776.95.L96 2016   613   C2016-900809-6
                                     C2016-900810-X

Fear the nutrition guru whose opinions don't change.
—Yoni Freedhoff, MD

"In 6 weeks, I lost 14 pounds of fat and gained 11 pounds of muscle. Everything fit better, I slept deeply, I woke rested, my anxious mind had substantially calmed itself, I had energy all day long, my skin was glowing, my eyes were bright, and I had the most amazing sense of well-being. I have always been skeptical of weight loss and nutrition programs, but can honestly say NOURISH was the missing piece of the puzzle that has changed my life." – *Pam Vorkapic*

"NOURISH gave me an entirely new perspective on healthy food and how it makes a difference in your well-being. The improved energy and stamina that I feel today, at age 61, are a direct result of applying the principles of NOURISH, and I am very thankful." – *Judd Gilks*

"Nourish changed my whole life. My marriage, finances, work relationships and my overall being all got better when my nutrition got better. A life changer for me." – *Charlene Wells*

"NOURISH will become your quintessential, go-to-guide to reclaiming your health and vitality through Cait's brilliantly comprehensive, relevant, and practical nutrition coaching. Eminently thoughtful and full of practical wisdom, NOURISH is a must read." – *Carey Dinkel*

"NOURISH: A system to learn and grow with—a life changer." – *Robert West*

"I am in my fourth, decade committed to public health as a registered nurse. Cait's knowledgeable, practical and straightforward nutritional coaching has improved my overall health by leaps and bounds." – *Virginia Marshall*, RN

"How we eat can change the world." – *Laura Easter*

For Lila

CONTENTS

FOREWORD

Cait's nutrition coaching focuses on the needs and lifestyle of each individual. Her advice is grounded in real-life sustainable recommendations that guide each person to choose the nutritious whole foods that work for them, at that time, in that moment or stage of their life. There are no lotions, potions, or magic pills. This is the real thing. An opportunity to get off of the diet merry-go round and choose health and vitality.

In responding to the needs of each person we are guided through behavioral change to truly optimize health and wellness by selecting the nutrient-rich foods that are right for us. This customization and use of real-life food and practices is what works. You can literally see people come to life in a matter of weeks.

Personally I have spent years following all the recommendations for health and weight loss or management. I've followed advice for reducing fat, lowering calorie intake, and increasing exercise. After years of trying to "do my best" and "work harder" I was exhausted and under nourished. Cait's coaching has taught me to use whole, nutrient-rich food and a balanced lifestyle to nourish my body and my life. Now, with ongoing training, I am using what I have learned with my own patients and seeing fantastic results.

NP Samantha Dalby, Nurse Practitioner
RN-EC, PHCNP, BscN, BA-Hons.

INTRODUCTION

CHAPTER ONE

Only the curious have something to find.
–Unknown

My Story

As I write this, I am 43. When I was in my teens, I wanted to fit into my custom equestrian riding boots. To do this, I tried a Diet Coke diet for three days, consuming nothing but cola and popcorn. I stopped the Diet Coke diet on day three when I was so weak and light-headed that I almost fell off my horse.

In my twenties, I continued my endeavours to be thin. I subsisted on a diet of these staples:

- coffee
- beer
- wine
- peas with rice
- pasta
- salad with non-fat dressing

In my thirties, and in particular pre-pregnancy, I ate more healthfully by North American standards:

- low fat
- whole grains
- lots of fruit and vegetables
- low calorie
- little red meat
- no butter
- no added salt

However, as I aged—especially after the birth of my daughter, Lila, in 2003 and after turning 35 in 2006—I did not see positive changes in my body composition (lean muscle mass to fat ratio) or my digestion. I could not sleep and I was depressed. I was fit from exercising, but my body fat was too high for how hard I exercised, my digestion was terrible, I was an insomniac, and I was discouraged.

In 2000, I was diagnosed with Lyme disease, ehrlichiosis and, babesiosis. As part of my healing protocol, I took a heavy-duty cocktail of antibiotics for six months. As a result, my Lyme disease (et al) was held at bay, but both the disease and the cure destroyed my digestive system. I was either too loose or I was constipated. I could not find a balance, even with lots of vegetables, fruits, water, and over-the-counter, fibre supplements.

In 2004, I changed careers. I left the equine industry and began building my fitness business, Custom Fit Vitality. I worked part-time in the evenings, as my days were spent with my daughter. In 2008, my fitness business broke wide open for me; I was working full time—60 plus hours per week. My enthusiasm for my work and my loyalty to my clients kept me upright. But my stress levels were diabolical, and it showed in my body composition. I was storing extra fat because I was so stressed, and I was over-exercising to deal with the stress and the extra fat. The only answer I could come up with, based on my research and knowledge at the time, was to eat less and work out more. I did a lot of faking it out in the world—especially in my fitness business. This was an exhausting front to maintain.

Behind the scenes, I did not sleep, because I was wired and tired from over-exercising and unintentionally starving myself. I lived on caffeine during the day to keep me up and red wine at night in order to bring myself down. Both the caffeine and the wine added to my insomnia, which was also fed by my overly active, anxious, monkey mind—a mind that would not shut off regardless of fatigue levels. I could not sleep. I was run down. My skin broke out and was dull and dry. I was sick a lot. My menstrual cycle was intense, with PMS and cramps. My body composition was not where I wanted it and I felt fat. My brain was on monkey-mind over-drive.

This was after years of diligent, healthy living, including eating whole grains, fruit, vegetables, lean protein, and non-fat dairy and giving up wheat. I ran five to eight kilometres, three to five days per week. I strength trained up to six days per week, with heavy weights and I allowed for recovery with days off every week. I also added in a steady yoga practice, for stress relief and flexibility. I meditated every morning for twenty minutes or more and I journaled for my busy monkey mind. And, I went to psychotherapy sessions.

After all of this healthy living on a consistent basis, I did not see positive changes in my body composition. I did not look or feel as fit as I actually was, I was not getting much for all that I was putting in, and I was tired of putting on the fa-cade of go-getter. I was maintaining my lean muscle mass, but my body would not release the layer of fat over the muscle, no matter how hard I worked my program. My digestion was still irregular. I still could not sleep, and my depression re-mained. Feeling poorly was frustrating, given my nature and my line of work. But instead of quitting—*how could I, given my career choice?*—I rallied. I decided to delve a bit deeper.

Surrounded by people looking to improve themselves with nutrition and fitness taught me that it doesn't matter how great we look, how much money we make or how full we stock our "fix-me-cupboards." When we are rotting from the inside out—when we have to fake it—we're never con-tent. We're worn out, starving, sexless, sleepless, and some-times, surly. We learn (or we don't) that "harder" in our work, our workouts and our world requires more, longer, earlier, and later which includes forsaking our relationships, our chil-dren and ultimately, ourselves. No matter how hard we lean in we don't fly. We're wind burned and grounded in the most prohibitive way. Then, exhausted from faking it, we go fetal behind the scenes. We learn (or we don't) that roaring around, full of purpose and passion, is as poor as aimlessly floating through life without a plan.

"Make me a superhero," a prospective client said to me one day, with her eyes sprung, lips full, breath hot and hon-eyed. She was that close to me—leaning in.

"A superhero?" I said.

"Yes! A superhero. I want to be faster, lighter and live forever! That is what I want. Can you help me?"

The potential client sitting across from me on the stark, white bench in my fitness studio was already a superhero. A successful entrepreneur, she'd zipped over for a lunch hour consult. A svelte, size four, she was married to a man who loved her with two kids, a McMansion, a cottage, a couple of imported SUVs, and multiple European and tropical holidays a year.

It was not enough. She wanted to be a superhero....

Later the same day, I sat across from another client who said, "I wish something in my fix-me-cupboard would work."

"What do you mean? What needs fixing?" I asked.

"Me," she said. "I need fixing. I am not happy."

"What aren't you happy with?"

"Me," she said, "I am not happy with me."

I could relate to both women... Curious by nature and determined to lead by example for my family and my clients, I remained hopeful that the answer to feeling better was out there somewhere.

Since 2009, my eating habits have changed a lot. This change in my diet started in earnest when my curiosity was piqued by the gluten-free craze. The research and the results people experienced amazed me! On every magazine cover, every talk show, the evening news, and confirmed by popular books from experts recommending grain-free diets, there were stories of people experimenting with a wheat-free life-style and feeling better. Inspired and excited to implement this change in my own diet, I could not wait to share this in-formation with my clients. As a result of this sharing, I have had many clients see huge changes just by eliminating gluten from their diets. (A client of mine wrote a grain-free cookbook, inspired by a Wheat-Free 21-Day Challenge I offered in 2011!)

But going wheat-free did not create the changes I wanted. And when I ate gluten-free products, I got a pounding headache and agonizing digestive issues. Upon reflection, I realized what I already knew as a trainer: any diet will create change. But the questions are:

Is the diet healthy?

Will results of the diet last?

The people I read about or knew who reaped the rewards of going gluten-free had great results because they were paying attention and eating more healthfully. But most people could not sustain their new routines for long.

I decided to take it a step further; I went completely grain-free.

Next, I added in more healthy fats. Today, my diet consists of 50 to 70 per cent healthy fats, comprised of things like: full-fat dairy (including 35 per cent heavy cream in my morning coffee), coconut oil, and at least half an avocado most days.

Out of necessity, I varied my fibre sources. If you quit grains, you have to find alternative fibre sources or you could experience a wide range of digestive issues, including constipation and diarrhea. Today, no matter what, I get at least 20 grams of fibre per day. As you will learn, fibre is one of the things around which you will base your daily nutrient rich intake for NOURISH. Fibre is one of the two NOURISH game changers.

The next big piece of the puzzle was getting my head around game changer number two: sugar. Even though I did not use table sugar and rarely ate junk food, I was unaware of how much my sugar and carbohydrate consumption was out of control. Sugar and carbohydrates from natural, healthy sources, including whole grains and fruits, were wreaking havoc on my whole system—especially fructose (fruit sugar). Learning how sugar affects my body and my mind is an education that continues for me still today. Now my daily sugar intake is less than 24 grams, and my husband and daughter have made positive changes around their sugar intake as well. For example, we are a juice-free household. Getting a handle on our sugar intake—both added and natural sugars—improved all facets of our wellness.

Exercise

I cut back on exercise and stopped distance running altogether. Instead, I came up with a training routine that works better for my body: high intensity,interval, strength training combined with sprinting once or twice a week, yoga, and Pilates. Today I work out three to four hours per week versus the seven to ten that I used to.

For me, experimenting with these changes—these decisions—helped me to understand even better this one simple concept: You cannot out-train a poor diet.

Even if you think your lifestyle is healthy by mainstream standards—*even if the whole world thinks you look great*—if you feel poorly, something is wrong. It does not matter how fit you think you are or how well you think you eat. If you feel like hell, it is time for a change.

NOURISH

Comprehensive and intensely personal, NOURISH captures the culmination of my research as a nutrition and fitness coach since 2004 for men and women, ranging in ages from tween to 75+. NOURISH does not discriminate; it is rooted in a platform of self-care and nutrition that combines commonly available, nutrient-rich food with a system I developed, called TAAP: Track, Assess, Adjust, Progress. The TAAP system teaches you how to hone in on your nutritional tipping points based on daily macronutrient consumption of protein, fats and carbohydrates and the two game changers: fibre and sugar. As a compass on the NOURISH program, you will rate the quality of four essential elements of your wellness which are: digestion, sleep, mood, energy.

NOURISH requires focus on two key questions:
What are you hungry for?
What are you getting for what you are eating?
You will also hear from the following people:

The Case Studies

The Correctional Officer: Justine knew that she was "skinny-fat" and she was frustrated about how to feed both herself and her family. Open-minded and quick to learn, Justine embraced healthier choices for herself and her loved ones. Upping her daily calorie allotment by including higher fat, low-sugar, fibre choices has given her back her life. Just 10 days into the NOURISH program, she felt more energized and alive.

The Grandmother: Learn from Bonnie about how she travels and continues to eat well while on the road to see her grandkids.

The Lifelong Dieter: Lucinda is a 60-year-old chronic dieter who finally stopped starving herself. She subsequently found herself healthier and happier.

The Retired Civil Servant: Instead of being a slave to diets, at 67 Abigail decided that she could improve her health by learning about which foods worked best for her.

The Soldier: Adam ate too low-calorie and was not feeding his brain with enough healthy fats. He could not sleep and he was depressed. Adam suffered from having very little energy and a scattered, foggy brain that made him have to fake it through his days. Food helped him to manage his Post Traumatic Stress Disorder (PTSD) and turned his life around.

The Entrepreneur: Weight was never an issue for Kelly. Kelly's problems were her overly active monkey mind and volatile digestive system. Finding her nutritional tipping points for protein, fats and carbohydrates and the two game changers, sugar and fibre, made all the difference. She now has more energy to care for her three children and run her new business.

The Retired IT: Kevin came to the NOURISH program with no complaints and a curious mind. He was open to experimenting with his nutrition in order to continue to age well and thrive as a grandfather and active golfer.

The Iron Woman Triathlete: Ruby, an ex-triathlete, woke up at 50 and thought, "What happened to my very fit self?" NOURISH helped Ruby get back her energy and a healthier body composition.

The Twenty Something: Avery shares how she now understands that exercising more and eating less were just making her skinny-fat.

The Doctor: Understanding all of the health issues that come with poor eating inspired Rebecca to look beyond traditional thinking. Healthy fats are now her new best friend.

The Hunter: Bill ate healthfully but was storing fat, his blood sugar plummets were a challenge, his cholesterol was high, and he couldn't sleep. Once he started eating enough protein, fats and fibre, he turned his life around for the better.

The Professional: Find out how Jessica kicked her diet soda habit for good and stopped using social gatherings as an excuse to overeat (or not to eat at all).

The Recovering Alcoholic: The aha moment for Dinah on the NOURISH program was discovering that her sugar habit had replaced her vodka habit. Once she realized she was addicted, she treated sugar like a drug and kicked the habit by managing her nutrition.

The Over-Exerciser: Tyson never had a weight issue, slept well and had no digestive issues. But he was hungry all the time and over-exercised to manage stress. Once he understood how natural sugars affected his hunger and he started eating more healthy fats, Tyson was able to cut back on exercise and calm his monkey mind.

The Teacher: Bethany found acceptance of her own body and she now encourages her tween daughters to do the same.

The Artist: Trina shares that change is a process and that old habits can become new, healthier ones.

The Librarian: After gastric bi-pass, Judith learned that choosing nutrient rich foods over diet foods created the road to wellness the worked best for her.

The Photographer: Evangeline learned that dieting and exercise would only take her so far on her fat loss journey. Her NOURISH epiphany: she was unintentionally *starving* herself! Evangeline made strides when she focused on nutrients instead of just calories.

The Food-Phobic, College Student: Vincent embraced how food could help him with his psychological disorder by studying how nutrient-rich foods improved his well-being compared to nutrient-dead, diet foods.

The Engineer: Jonathon gave up his Friday-night beer binges for more avocados—and he's never felt better.

The Tween Girl: Louise gave up juice, crackers and granola bars to find more self-confidence and tame the "hangries" (hungry and angry!).

The Tween Boy: Benjamin conquered his digestive issues and chronic headaches and regained his love of sports.

Back to You

Forget about fridge lists, forbidden foods, and skipping cake on your birthday. It's time to reclaim nutritional and energetic prosperity with the proven solution: NOURISH—a platform of wellness designed specifically for y-o-u. Are you ready to begin?

CHAPTER TWO

There are only two mistakes one can make along the road to truth;
not going all the way, and not starting.
–Buddha

Are You Nutritionally Bankrupt?

Is it possible that you are both overfed and under NOUR-ISHed? Could you be unintentionally starving yourself? Yes, yes and yes!

The diet industry cheats us with short-lived fixes and fantastical promises. We live on fast, cheap, and easy food, or we consume nutrient-dead health food that does not nourish us. Because of this, many of us are overfed, under NOURISHed and hungry; we are nutritionally bankrupt.

NOURISH is about wherever you are right now, at this moment. You may be: over-fat, under-fat, in shape, out of shape, on the healthy-lifestyle wagon or totally off it.

I remind my clients that we have our whole lives to get it right—whatever works best for us as individuals. We are all a work in progress. Nutrition continues to evolve, and yet the basic principle remains the same: healthy food is nutrient-rich food. Embrace this simple fact and you will succeed on the NOURISH program.

As you move forward, keep an open, curious mind. It is time to discover how to get off the magical misery tour of what and when to eat. We may be shaking up what you currently know about food in terms of why, when, and what to eat. Here are some myths to tuck away for the time being. If you choose, you can always come back to them if you believe that they still serve you. They are not going anywhere.

Myths

- You must eat breakfast.
- You must eat mini-meals every three to four hours.
- A calorie is a calorie.
- You must eat three meals a day.
- You must not eat after dinner.
- You must eat low fat to be, or to stay, low fat.
- The calories-in-versus-calories-out myth that we can burn off extra calories with exercise.
- To burn fat, you need long, slow distance (LSD) cardio.
- Red meat is bad for you.
- Vegetarianism is the wave of the future.
- The 80/20 rule: You can eat well 80 per cent of the time and do what you want the other 20 per cent.
- Cheat days—that one day a week you can eat whatever you want.
- You can "run off" your fries and milk shake—you can out-train a poor diet.

Say Goodbye To:

- dieting
- starvation
- bingeing
- cheat days
- yo-yo dieting

Any diet will create change. But ask yourself:

Is the diet healthy?
Will the results of the diet last?

With NOURISH, you are about to discover how to get off the magical misery tour of what and when to eat. You will learn the TAAP system: TRACK, ASSESS, and ADJUST, to PROGRESS. TAPP is the toolkit designed to help you develop the nutritional skills, self-care routines, and mindset you need to reclaim nutritional and energetic prosperity. With TAAP, you will take control of your health and life in a balanced and positive way. Through TAAP, you will discover your own nutritional tipping points to design a customized foundation for your health and wellness. Throughout NOURISH, you will use your answers to four key ASSESSment questions as your compass to find your nutritional tipping points:

- How is my digestion?
- How is my sleep?
- How is my mood?
- How is my energy level?

To enhance these four essential elements of your health, NOURISH will teach you to focus on asking two basic questions: What am I hungry for? What am I getting for what I am eating?

The Ground Rules for NOURISH:
- Read each lesson carefully, and take notes.
- Reread each lesson carefully, and take more notes.
- Participate fully—do the work.

That's it. It's pretty simple.

Now, let's discover your nutritional tipping points and get ready to master NOURISH—your personalized nutrition system that delivers unbeatable, sustainable results.

CHAPTER THREE

> *The expectations of life depend upon diligence;*
> *the mechanic that would perfect his work must first sharpen his tools.*
> —Confucius

Before You Start: NOURISH Tools

A successful journey requires the right tools. Here are the tools you need for NOURISH.

1. A nutrient tracking app: Down load a free, nutrient tracking app. You will use the app to TRACK your nutrients. Notice I did not say calorie counter—I said *nutrient* tracker. Throughout NOURISH you will use the weekly dietary summary reports provided by the app to ASSESS and AD-JUST as part of the TAAP system.

Here is a list of free, nutrient trackers:

fatsecret.com

myfitnesspal.com

loseit.com

sparkpeople.com

2. A kitchen scale: You will need a digital kitchen scale to accurately measure your food. If you do not have a kitchen scale for weighing food, buy one. You can purchase a scale for around $25.- that is about the size and profile of an iPad mini and needs to live on your kitchen counter.

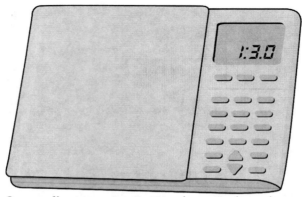

Some diets suggest measuring portion sizes with body parts like the size of your palm for meat or your thumb for a piece of cheese (or the size of your appetite). I wish measuring with body parts were reliable. It is not. This is the lazy person's way of not taking responsibility for the effects of how the foods you eat either build you up or break you down. Because, make no mistake—everything you eat does one or the other. Believe it or not, too much healthy food can make you cranky, fat, and hyper just like a candy bar or an entire pizza—whether it is loaded with veggies or not.

3. A cloth tape measure: You will use a cloth tape to measure sites on your body at the start middle and end of NOURISH. An explanation of where and what you need to record can be found in the **Your Starting Point** chapter.

4. Body fat measuring callipers: You will need a set of body fat measuring callipers. Understanding your body fat percentage is key to managing your health and wellness. You will use the callipers to find out how much of your weight on the scale is lean mass (blood, bones, organs, muscles, water, etc.) and how much of your body weight is actual body fat. Your body fat percentage number is based on your gender, your age, your weight on the scale and the subcutaneous fat measurements you will take using body fat callipers. You can order your callipers for about $35.- online at amazon.com or amazon.ca, or you can pick them up at GNC.

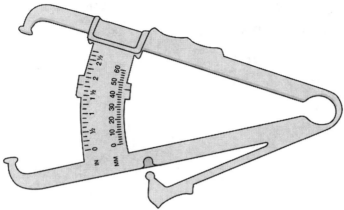

5. A body weight scale. A regular bathroom scale is fine and digital is best. You will just use the scale to find your body weight at the beginning, middle and end of NOURISH to help calculate your body fat percentage.

6. A trusted friend or partner to take your photographs at the beginning, middle and end of NOURISH.

Optional Tools: A streaks or goal tracker app on your smart phone to track your consistency and a journal or notebook to record your progress.

READER'S NOTES:

PART I:
Acknowledge

CHAPTER FOUR

There are no facts, only interpretations.
–Friedrich Nietzsche

Over Fed and Under NOURISHed

As a society, whether we are over or underfed, many of us are under NOURISHed. We are full of drink and yet dehydrated. Everything in our closets is tight or hanging off us like wet towels. The answer to the question *Why don't we do better when we know better?* is an elusive one. In many ways, this simple question has provided me with job security. As a nutrition and fitness coach, the self-sabotage I see in my clients has kept me in business since 2004. In my work, I see a pattern of habits contributing to the nutritional undermining of hundreds of people on a regular basis. This has been the focus of my research for over a decade. Here are some facts about my clients:

- The median age of my clients is 42.
- Many of my clients are parents and some are grandparents.
- Almost all of the people I coach work outside of the home.
- Most of these men and women are stressed out…

A reputable naturopath could diagnose many of my clients as suffering from adrenal fatigue. This often overwhelming fatigue can be brought on by mental, emotional, or physical stress. Some of these people are exhausted, quick-tempered, overly emotional, uninspired, not thinking clearly, sleepless and living on the edge.[1]

Prospective clients call me as a last resort, after they have tried: dieting, bingeing and purging, learn-to-run workshops, women or men only circuit training clubs, diet groups, tai chi, extreme exercise videos and classes, community exercise in the park, gardening clubs, book clubs, starvation, and endless amounts of self-loathing.

How many of the above have you tried?

These people spent money on gym memberships that they did not use. They swore to commit their spouses and kids to family passes at the local gym and they never went. These were people who loaded-up on late-night, infomercial exercise DVD's, they asked for treadmills for their anniversaries and they gave up all the foods they love—all to look and feel better. Many of them did not have cake on their birthdays. Or, they ate cake shamefully, alone, after everyone had gone to bed...with a pint of ice cream to wash it down. These were men and women who drank red wine in excess because of the "health benefits," or they sipped vodka and soda (no cranberry juice—too many carbs) and light beer at functions, as wallflowers, as far away from the buffet as possible. Or, they stationed themselves at the buffet and once they started eating, they had no brakes—they could not stop.

Some of these examples include people who did not sleep and did not have sex. They resisted being photographed; they would not wear a bathing suit. They insisted that they had it all under control. That is, until they didn't.

In my initial consults with prospective clients, I find that people have four, main issues in common. They experience one or more of the following:

- digestion distress
- sleeplessness
- monkey mind chaos
- low or unmanageable energy levels

After telling their stories, first, there was a desire to change; then, out came the arsenal of excuses. And the biggest excuse people shared was aging...

Aging Statistics to Ruminate On

Starting in our twenties, our metabolism, which is responsible for all of the life sustaining physical and chemical processes in the body, begins to slow down.[2] If we change nothing, we could see a potential gain of non-essential body fat. This extra fat is often referred to as the "middle-aged spread." Further, after the age of thirty, we lose three to five per cent of our lean muscle mass per decade. The good news is that it is not old age but *lifestyle* that determines this for us.[3] The key to aging well is intelligent nutrition, stress management and purposeful exercise.

When new clients say they do not have time for self-care, I ask them, "Who will look after everything when you fall?"

The burden of the sick falls on the healthy and the details of death and dying are for the living. I believe that the hand of the universe opens wider for people who help other people. But, we have to put the oxygen mask on ourselves first. Everything about life gets better when we practice self-care that serves us. Again, a foundation of hydration, nutrient rich foods, sleep, and thoughtful, intentional exercise is key.

CHAPTER FIVE

First and foremost, you have to know why you want to do this.
—Laura Easter

Get Over Your Self. Get Started!

Tough love? Maybe. I tell my clients, when they offer their arsenal of excuses: *Begin. Just start.* Yes, you may be: fat, tired, overwhelmed, busy, scared, scrawny, weak, uncoordinated, not naturally athletic, broke or slightly broken...

And, you may not be what you used to be in high school. Let me tell you this: *Nobody cares!* And, in the most compassionate way, that is true. Here is why:

> Many of us are addicted to our excuses in one way or another.
>
> Everyone has issues that are in plain sight or are hidden behind the scenes.
>
> Each one of us craves support and guidance on the path to wellness.
>
> Most of us learned what we know about how to feed our bodies from our parents or caretakers.

The questions are:

> How much did yours know?
>
> How healthy were (are) your mentors?

Are you curious about your nutrition but overwhelmed about where to start? The take-away nugget is that there is no need to be embarrassed. Have you ever had a big project that you needed to dig into but instead of starting, you kept coming up with a long list of to dos that took precedence?

> When I have more money...
>
> After I make this call...
>
> When I have more free time...
>
> After this TV show is over...

When so-and-so gets home to help me...

YOU are the project, and your excuses are just noise when it comes to health and wellness:

Once I lose some weight...

After my cruise...

As soon as the holidays are over...

Just as soon as the kids go off to school...

If I could get my spouse on board...

In my experience as a coach, all of the above might look like laziness or procrastination but all of those excuses stem from one thing: fear. Some of the fear comes from the unknown. For example, who are we if we're not constantly trying to fix ourselves? No matter what, there is always something that can anchor us down into the abyss of poor health if we let it. Cut the cord, saw off the chain, turn down the volume on the justifications in your head and get going. It's time to get over your self, and get started!

My first excuse was "I don't cook when my husband doesn't cook for me." I knew that I made the right choice in calling Cait when she said, "What are you, five-years-old?"

–Dinah, NOURISH client

CHAPTER SIX

The secret of all victory lies in the organization of the non-obvious.
—Marcus Aurelius

The TAAP System: TRACK, ASSESS, ADJUST, PROGRESS

The first question I ask my clients when they say they eat well is "How do you know?" They look at me as if I'm crazy.

But then they say, "Well, I guess I don't."

My response is "You need to."

Why TAAP?

Like anything, the TAAP system must be practiced to become a lifelong habit.

TAAP is the most important component to NOURISH. When I first started the nutrient TRACKking required for NOURISH, it seemed labour intensive. But, like anything that is truly worthwhile, it takes practice to be good at it. Practice and you'll become proficient. TRACKing is a critical tool to help us make positive change.
—Bonnie, NOURISH client

Think about other areas in your life that you paid closer attention to and that improved incrementally. It may have been: selling or finding a new house, looking for a new job, improving your finances, making time for date nights with your partner, creating more family time or, craving more YOU time.

TRACKing helps us focus on learning what works for us nutritionally and what does not. It is through keeping TRACK that you will discover your own nutritional tipping points. On a scale of one to 10, you will rate the quality of your digestion, your sleep, your mood and your energy levels. You will use your answers as your compass.

When I started TRACKing and ASSESSing all my food, I couldn't believe how little I was eating. No wonder I felt weak. This made my job tough, as I run after children all day! It took me about two weeks to start feeling a change mentally and physically. And, I finally regained the energy I needed for successful workouts; I could push through, unlike before.

–Avery, NOURISH client

For someone who is just starting out, I cannot stress this enough: read labels and TRACK, ASSESS, and ADJUST, to PROGRESS. Concentrate and keep a record of how you feel. And, I mean every-thing—energy, mood, sex drive. When I stray from what I should be eating, I notice how it has affected me as soon as I get back on the straight and narrow. It is absolutely amazing how much better I feel. That is such a motivator for continuing. And, like NOURISH teaches, you cannot know unless you TRACK.

–Constance, NOURISH client

It is time to foster habits that truly serve you. It's time to start. Are you ready to TAAP?

CHAPTER SEVEN

Acknowledge What Is

As part of the TRACK, ASSESS, ADJUST and PROGRESS (TAAP) system, decide where you see yourself right now in the following poem:

Autobiography in Five Short Chapters
–By Portia Nelson

1.
I walk down the street.
There is a deep hole in the sidewalk.
I fall in.
I am lost I am hopeless.
It isn't my fault.
It takes forever to find a way out.

2.
I walk down the same street.
There is a deep hole in the sidewalk.
I pretend I don't see it.
I fall in again.
I can't believe I am in the same place.
But it isn't my fault.
It still takes a long time to get out.

3.
I walk down the same street.
There is a deep hole in the sidewalk.
I see it is there.
I still fall in ... it's a habit.
My eyes are open.

I know where I am.
It is my fault.
I get out immediately.

4.
I walk down the same street.
There is a deep hole in the sidewalk.
I walk around it.

5.
I walk down another street.

Complete this sentence: I see myself in chapter_____

Why? How do you know?
What will be different this time around?
Today's Date: DD_____MM_____YYYY_____

I'm in chapter one. As for what I want more of in my life, I want more of a sense of control and balance, as well as purpose. [I want] to be happy and content. Essentially, I want to come out of chapter one an even better person than I was before my struggle began.
–Vincent, NOURISH client

For programs like this, people often jump to the standard goals: You want to lose weight for the wedding. You want to train for a half-marathon. You want to lose weight to keep the spark alive in our relationship. You get the idea…

At Custom Fit, I do not offer things like wedding-party boot camps. Just looking good in those dresses and tuxes for one day is not a good enough goal. Soon after the wedding, you will experience a letdown that leaves you feeling hollow and, ultimately, like you need fixing again. The reason? The "why", being thinner or more "buff," was simply not big enough. Instead, put down the instant gratification mindset of *Fix Me Now!* Get clear on why you are doing NOURISH.

It may be that you want to eat healthier so you can conceive because you are too skinny or too fat to get or to stay pregnant. Perhaps, you want the energy and mental patience to play with and enjoy your grandchildren. Maybe you want to proactively prevent lifestyle diseases that run in your family or, you want to get off medications that give you dangerous side effects. It could be that you want to rekindle your passion for life (be specific).

Your next assignment is to get really clear on what you want more of in your life. What is it?

Finish this statement: **I want more...**Think about it. Take your time.

List three specific reasons why you want to do this program:

List three reasons why *now* is the right time and you are ready to commit to yourself:

List three things you will do to create positive change in your health:

Complete these sentences:

By the end of NOURISH, in 12 weeks, on_____(date)

   I will feel...

   I will look...

   I will be...

   Because...

Now you can start to develop simple, yet comprehensive, intentions, practices, and goals that will sustain, NOURISH, and bless the venture and the joys of daily living—*for you.*

CHAPTER EIGHT

Wisdom begins in wonder.
—Socrates

Your Starting Point

First, you need to acknowledge your starting point. Even if you want to dive right in, you need to acknowledge where you are today. Now is the time to ask the four key ASSESS-ment questions.

Rate each one on a scale of 1 to 10 (1 = poor; 10 = excellent).

How is your digestion? Why?
How is your sleep? Why?
How is your mood? Why?
How is your energy level? Why?
Today's Date: DD_____MM_____YYYY_____

To establish your starting point, you will take your:

- photographs
- measurements
- metrics
- and you will choose a target article of clothing

Look at your calendar and mark down your dates for metrics and photographs.

Start Date: DD_____MM_____YYYY_____
Six Weeks Date: DD_____MM_____YYYY_____
12 Weeks Date: DD_____MM_____YYYY_____

Your Photographs

First, find someone to take your photographs. These photos will be an integral part of benchmarking your PROGRESS. You will be grateful to have them as a reference sooner than you think. Have someone take four, full body photos of you from the following angles: front, left, right, and rear. Wear a bathing suit or make sure to wear something as form fitting as possible. And, do not wear all black! Your Johnny Cash days are behind you. You will take your photographs again at six weeks and then again at 12 weeks.

When I meet with clients for their six weeks metrics appointments, it is not the data of the metrics or their weight on the scale that convinces them that they are making progress. Even if they feel better and look healthier, it is the changes that they see in the photographs that are the most compelling. Seeing really is believing and the full body photographs don't lie.

Your Measurements

Next, record your measurements at the sites on your body listed below with a cloth measuring tape. You will do this today, at six weeks and again at 12 weeks. (Make sure to write down the six and 12 weeks dates right now so you are organized.)

Note: The shoulder circumference measurement is taken at the widest point, with the arms hanging at the sides and the shoulders relaxed.

Note: If you choose, you can measure any other part of your abdomen you wish to record. As a point of reference, measure the distance up or down from the belly button (circle one, so you'll remember). Most people chose one to three inches above or below the belly button (or both) and measure the circumference to obtain this additional measurement.

Using the cloth measuring tape, measure and record the following areas on your body:

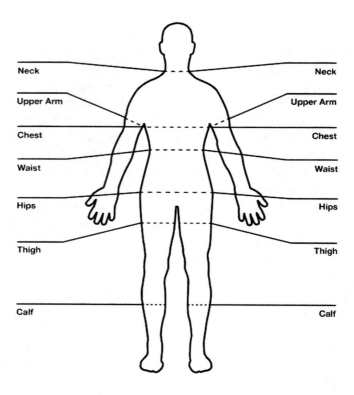

Measurement Chart (tape)				
Site on body	Start Date:	6 weeks Date:	12 weeks Date:	Totals +/-
Bust/Chest				
Ribcage (women only)				
6" below belly button				
Hips (widest point)				
Left thigh (top)				
Left knee (top)				
Left calf (widest point)				
Right thigh (top)				
Right knee (top)				
Right calf (widest point)				
Left arm (top of bicep)				
Right arm (top of bicep)				
Shoulders (widest point)				
Neck				
Optional: measure inches above or below belly button " above " below				

A Note About the Scale

For the purposes of this program, you will take your body weight on the scale and use it as part of your metrics. To calculate your body fat, you will use your weight and your age. To calculate your caloric ranges, you will use your weight, age and activity level.

That is the whole purpose of weighing yourself on the scale—that is it.

The goal of NOURISH is not (necessarily) to get lighter on the scale. It is about getting healthier on the inside. This can show up different ways on the scale. For example, if you gain lean muscle mass, you might end up heavier than when you started the program. But if you lose body fat during the process, you could end up smaller in body and clothing size.

The scale will lie to you; it can make you crazy. Here are some reasons the scale can be inaccurate:

You are dehydrated (making you lighter on the scale).

You are constipated (making you heavier on the scale).

You have been traveling and are retaining water (heavier).

You are experiencing PMS (heavier).

You had a very salty meal the night before (heavier).

You just worked out (lighter).

You just drank a litre of water (heavier).

You are *gaining* muscle and muscle weighs more than fat (heavier).

You are *losing* muscle and muscle weighs more than fat (lighter).

Any of the above, plus endless other factors, can cause the scale to make you happy or depressed at any given moment. Instead, use the four ASSESSment questions as your daily guide: How is your digestion? How is your sleep? How is your mood? How is your energy level?

Just jump ahead to the **Case Studies** section and read about the people who changed their body composition for the better (and their lives) without seeing the scale budge at all. Imagine how discouraged they would have been if they kept jumping on and off the scale, at random, throughout the program. It does not serve you to weigh here and there and then get discouraged by the number that you see on the scale. STAY OFF THE SCALE. Weigh yourself at the start, the middle and at the end of NOURISH.

Your Body Fat Metrics

Next, it is time to figure out your body fat percentage. How much of you is actual body fat, compared to how much of you is lean mass? Your lean mass includes your bones, blood, organs, muscle, and both essential and non-essential body water. (Did you know that body is made up of 60 per cent water[4]?) Understanding your body fat and where you fit in on the body fat categories table is one of the tools you will use to gauge your health and wellness.

In my experience, the easiest, and most reliable tool on the market today is the body fat calliper. You will use the Jackson/Pollock Seven Calliper Method to establish your body fat percentage. You can learn to test yourself on five of the seven required skin-fold areas. A trusted friend or partner can do the two you cannot reach on your own (the triceps area on the back of your arm and in between your shoulder blades for the subscapular measurement). Instructions on how to take the skin-fold measurements are included with your callipers. Practice on yourself multiple times to get the feel for the callipers, and ask the same person to help you each time you measure. Also, always measure (and weigh) at the same time of day.

Know that all measurements taken for NOURISH are *estimates*. Measuring like this is not a perfect science and it does not need to be! For NOURISH, we are using your measurements as tools to ASSESS your PROGRESS. The measurement process is not an exact science. The most important aspect of measuring is that the person doing so is consistent.

To calculate your body fat percentage, use an online body fat calculator like one of these:

> http://www.linear-software.com/online.html
> http://www.free-online-calculator-use.com/skin-fold-test.html
> http://www.exrx.net/Calculators/BodyComp.html

Instructions for using online, body fat calculators:

- Select male or female and double check to make sure the gender is correct. (Gender makes a difference in body fat calculations!)
- Enter your age and weight from the scale.
- Use the Jackson/Pollock Seven Calliper Method.
- Enter in your measurement numbers for each of the seven skin-fold areas.

- Press calculate.
- Record all of your data below for future reference.

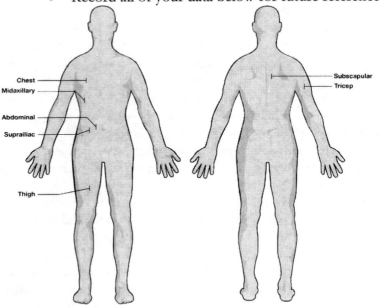

Measurement Chart (callipers)				
Site	Measurement #1 Date:	Measurement #2 Date:	Measurement #3 Date:	Totals +/-
Chest				
Abs				
Thigh				
Tricep				
Subscapular				
Suprailiac				
Midaxillary				
Weight				

What Do Your Metrics Mean?

Take a look at the body fat categories table below to see which category you fit in, based on your body fat percentage results.

Body Fat Categories		
Category	Women (% fat)	Men (% fat)
Essential Fat	10–13	2–5
Athletic	14–20	6–13
Fit	21–24	14–17
Acceptable	23–31	18–25
Obese	32+	26+

Where do you fit in on the table above? What do you think about your results? Surprised? Nervous? Disgusted? Relieved?

First, wherever you ended up, do not panic! You have taken the first step to proactively taking charge of your health. If, based on the chart, you think you are too lean or overly fat, remember, this is not an exact science! I have both male and female clients who are very lean with body fat calculations that put them into or below the essential fat category by a point or two. These people are healthy and have plenty of energy and lean muscle mass. I also have clients who register in the obese category who are hardly ever sick and who work out regularly. And, to be clear, I have clients at both ends of the spectrum who are not well, are sick all the time and have multiple health issues. I have clients who show up in the fit or athletic range who are anything but!

This is why when I coach a client, I look at *the whole person* to make sure we get the *whole picture*. It is imperative that you do the same thing as you coach yourself through NOURISH. This is why I ask you to ASSESS your digestion, your sleep, your mood and your energy levels. And, this is why those photographs I asked you to take are so important! It is also why I asked you to answer the ASSESSment questions before you started. Acknowledging and TAAPing are the keys to your success.

Next ...Choose a Target Article of Clothing

You need to choose a target article of clothing that you can try on weekly as a marker of your PROGRESS. Think of your target article of clothing as another metric in your AS-SESSment toolkit. For men, it could be a pair of jeans or dress pants with a smaller-sized waist, or a dress shirt that you have trouble buttoning up. For women, it could be a blouse, a pair of jeans, or a dress. Some people choose a bathing suit. Either pull something out of your closet you have not been able to wear for a while or go shopping. Whatever you choose, do not try your outfit on every day! Try it on weekly, on the same day, and at the same time. What is your target article of clothing? Why did you choose this? What day will you try on your target article of clothing?

Note: Do not "shop" up a size in your closet. Once something is too big or doesn't suit you anymore, donate or toss it!

You need *all* of this initial data to establish your starting point:

- your answers to all of the ASSESSment questions
- your photographs
- your cloth tape measurements
- your body fat and lean mass calculations
- and your target outfit

This data along with the answers to the four key AS-SESSment questions are crucial parts of the TAAP system. Just using the scale is not enough to measure your health and wellness. In a few shorts weeks you will be glad that you took the time to clearly establish your starting point.

Got Belly Fat?

Belly fat is code for visceral fat. Visceral fat surrounds our internal organs and increases our risk of many health issues and diseases including, heart disease, diabetes and stroke. Genetics, lifestyle and poor nutritional choices are linked to excess belly fat.[5] In my research, I have seen many clients who come for coaching after years of eating a low calorie, low fat, carbohydrate laden diet—both simple and complex—and who carry extra belly fat. This includes clients who live on whole grains and copious amounts of fruits and vegetables. As soon as they make the change to nutrient rich, lower sugar, higher fibre choices, they begin to lose belly fat, improve their digestion, sleep better, their moods level off and their energy levels increase or are more manageable.

Next, it is time to TRACK your food and water for three days so you can ASSESS where you are starting nutritionally. Then you can make ADJUSTments from an educated place and make PROGRESS by discovering your nutritional tipping points.

CHAPTER NINE

Show me what you eat and I will show you what you are.
—Jean Anthelme Brillat-Savarin

First, Change Nothing and TRACK

After establishing your physical starting point, it is time to figure out where you are with your nutrition. Use your nutrient tracking app to log everything you put into your mouth. The TRACK part of TAAP is the first key to figuring out what you have been getting for what you have been eating.

And the first lesson is to change nothing.

Again, acknowledging your starting points physically and nutritionally is essential. You could easily skip ahead, jump right in, and start making changes to your diet. Right now. Today. But NOURISH offers a thinking person's journey to wellness. Use the nutrient tracking app to help you record your food for three days (and throughout the entire 12 weeks of NOURISH and beyond). A pen and paper will not do. The nutrient tracking app gathers the nutrient data from your food for you. Collecting this nutritional information is critical in order to ASSESS and ADJUST so you can make PROGRESS. You need to see what you have been getting for what you have been eating to understand where you need to go with your nutrition.

If I gave you a fridge list and told you exactly what to eat and when, you might do it for a while. And, if you had been eating a diet of nutrient dead foods or unintentionally starving yourself, you might begin to feel better. The body responds quickly to nutrient rich foods that serve it. But what would you have learned? Why would you feel better? What specific changes worked for you, and which did not?

You cannot know unless you TRACK and TRACKing is useless unless you ASSESS.

You must establish a clear picture of where you are starting from in order to fully understand the changes you will make. For three days, just track your food. When I say food, I mean everything that goes in your mouth. TRACK your food so you can collect all of the nutritional information you need in the dietary summary provided by the nutrient tracking app. After you TRACK for three days, you will review your dietary summary and ASSESS how you are doing. You'll ask, "What am I getting for what I am eating?"

Then, as you read, reread and learn the lessons in NOURISH, you will begin to incorporate them into your daily nutrient intake by making ADJUSTments to your diet. And, you will continue to TRACK and ASSESS.

And, then, you will PROGRESS. You will begin to ask (and answer) the question, *What am I hungry for?*

I promise that TRACKing your food on the nutrition tracking app becomes less cumbersome as you progress through NOURISH. As you enter your regular foods, the app remembers them for you. This encourages you to stick to nutrient rich foods, because they are already entered and you know how they work nutritionally for you—or do not.

Understand right now that healthy food is healthy food and that healthy people eat the same healthy food over and over again—it's that simple. I cannot stress this enough.

For now, for the first three days of TRACKing your food, just keep eating the way you always have. You need this information as a baseline to measure PROGRESS. Perhaps you have been eating too few calories. Maybe you need more protein or your healthy fat consumption is low. It could be that you are eating too much fibre and robbing your body of nutrition!

You cannot know unless you TRACK. And then you need to ASSESS so you can ADJUST from an educated place based on what you learn in the NOURISH lessons.

Eat the way you always have, just be sure to TRACK it. Anything that goes into your mouth—TRACK it. A relief? Annoyed? It doesn't matter. Have faith and TRACK.

After TRACKing for three days, you will review your detailed report on your nutrient tracking app to see your averages for your calories, the macronutrients protein, fats and carbohydrates and the two game changers fibre and sugar. Nutrient trackers have a lot of data on them! Do not get distracted. Again, for NOURISH, you will focus on your water consumption, your total calories and the three macronutrients— protein, fat and carbohydrates. You will also learn your nutritional tipping points for the two game changers, fibre and sugar. You will use your answers to the four ASSESSment questions as your compass: How is your digestion? How is your sleep? How is your mood? How is your energy?

Depending on the app you choose, your food log summary will look similar to NOURISH client Justine's food log. Below is an example of what a single day looked like for Justine on her first week of NOURISH: (A reminder that for NOURISH, you are focusing on the macronutrients protein, fat and carbohydrate and the two game changers fibre and sugar. For Justine's log, I have taken out all of the other data on the nutrient tracker to focus on the elements of NOURISH. When you look at your food logs, do not get distracted by the other data on your nutrient tracker. Just focus on what you need for this program.)

Sample Food Log	Prot (g)	Fat (g)	Sat (g)	Carbs (g)	Sugar (g)	Fibre (g)	Cals (kcal)
Breakfast							
Protein Shake 1 scoop (35g)	26	2.5	1	3	2	1	140
Frozen Mixed Berries 1 cup	1	0	0	17	11	3	70
Skim of Nonfat Milk (Calcium Fortified) 1 cup	8.4	0.44	0.289	11.98	11.98	0	86
Total	35.4	2.94	1.289	31.98	24.98	4	296
Lunch							
Skinless Chicken Breast 1/2 breast, bone and skin removed	27.25	1.46	0.389	0	0	0	130
Dinner							
Snacks/Other							
Grapes (Red or Green) European Type Varieties such as Thompson Seedless) 1 cup, seedless	1.15	0.26	0.086	28.96	24.77	1.4	110
Protein Bar 1 bar (60g)	21	8	3	21	1	17	210
Total	22.15	8.26	3.086	49.96	25.77	18.4	320
Total	84.8	12.66	4.764	81.94	50.75	22.4	746

It is very helpful to know where you stand in terms of your nutrient numbers before you start learning about where you "should" be. Do not underestimate the task of changing nothing first—it is invaluable to the learning process of NOURISH and figuring out what works for you.
–Kelly, NOURISH client

TRACK Your Water Consumption
Along with TRACKing your food, it is very important that you drink enough water daily. Properly hydrating yourself is part of a healthy lifestyle. Remember that our bodies are on average 60 per cent water. I recommend that my clients drink at least 64 ounces of water before three or four o'clock every day. If you practice drinking all of your water by three or four o'clock each day, you won't be up all night going to the bathroom. Water apps are genius. It may sound ridiculous, but if you TRACK your water on an app, the app keeps you accountable and timely with your water intake. Sometimes we

need a little nagging from an outside source to get things done!

Water Helps Us:

- lubricate our joints
- regulate our body temperature
- maintain blood volume
- prevent brain fog
- stay energized
- rid ourselves of non-essential body water (think sock lines and puffy eyes)[6]

Are You Chronically Dehydrated?

Think about a houseplant that is very dry. When it is finally watered, the water rushes out through the bottom. If you are not used to hydrating yourself regularly, you will pee a lot for the first couple of days on NOURISH. This will pass. You may revert to old habits and find yourself once again dehydrated, or you may allow yourself to quit because you *just can't drink all that water*, or you think *it's a chore*. That's okay! Just restart. **I repeat: it is very important that you drink enough water daily.**

Water Tips

Upon rising, drink eight ounces of water as soon as your feet hit the floor. Do your best to drink your water between feedings. This is much easier on the digestive system and produces less gas and bloating. Plus, when it's time to eat, you want to fill up with nutrients, not water. This is especially true if you are having issues with getting in enough calories through the day. You can add lemon, cucumber, lime, ginger, or mint to flavour your water. Get creative! Drink hot water or hot water and lemon and, add in a touch of cayenne pepper for an extra kick. Try drinking your water extra cold or try drinking it room temperature and everything in between. Find what water temperature is best for you. Drink herbal teas.

Add greens to your water. (Greens are a powdered drink supplement that you can add to water to increase our daily micronutrients. You can find greens at health food stores. Make sure to read the labels before you buy. Choose greens that are free from artificial ingredients.)

Also, you can count the water that you drink if you use protein shakes. Try adding twice the water to make the shake less sweet tasting and to increase your daily water intake. You can TAAP to see how the caffeine in tea and coffee affects your body.

Some studies suggest that caffeine is dehydrating. However, there is new research that suggests caffeine is not dehydrating because of the water content in coffee and tea.[7] Again, you cannot know unless you TRACK, ASSESS, and ADJUST as required. For example, I can drink two, eight ounce cups of coffee with 35 per cent heavy cream every morning without issue. If I consume more than two cups of coffee per day, my digestion gets too loose. If I drink coffee after one o'clock PM, I have trouble sleeping. I TAAP to figure this out. I do count the water in my coffee towards my total daily intake but because I exercise and my coaching work requires a lot of talking (which is dehydrating), I find that I need more than three litres per day. This means, I drink my coffee before noon and I drink an additional three litres of water by three or four o'clock every day. Note: Alcohol does not count towards your daily hydration goals!

Winter Hydration

Staying hydrated takes planning. This can be especially true in colder climates. During the warmer months we reach for our water bottles more often. Once it gets cold, sometimes we don't feel thirsty. My number-one tip for drinking more water in the winter is to drink broth or stock. Vegetable, chicken, or beef broth are good this time of year and homemade stock is nutrient rich. Add your favourite, savoury seasonings, and warm-up as you stay hydrated all day long.

For the next three days, TRACK your food and water. That's it. After three full days of TRACKing, you will start to learn about what the information you have TRACKed means when you ASSESS your food logs.

I would like to say tracking water is easy, but it takes practice. You get going in your day, and before you know it, your day is half over and you have not even had one glass of water. You have to have a system.
–Bill, NOURISH client

CHAPTER TEN

What are you getting for what you are eating?
—Cait Lynch

Check In and ASSESS your Food Logs

(Note: Before reading this chapter, make sure you have tracked your food and water for three days.)

You have tracked your food and water for three days now. Are you learning anything? Before you ASSESS your food log report, let's ASSESS a day of Justine's food log from her first week of TRACKing.

Take a look at Justine's calories first. Based on Justine's age, weight, and her body fat metrics, her Basal Metabolic Rate (BMR) is 1600 calories per day. The BMR is the baseline number of calories from nutrient-rich food Justine needs to consume daily in order to survive. (You will calculate your BMR in the **A Calorie is Not a Calorie** chapter.) With an average of just 1184 calories per day, this means that Justine did not meet her baseline, BMR, daily caloric requirements. No wonder her energy was so low! Also, as soon as Justine learned about healthy fats, she discovered that her daily average for fats was very low. Justine's carbohydrate intake was reasonable, but her protein levels were a bit high, given that she was not exercising. She would not have known these things unless she TRACKed and ASSESSed her food. Because Justine wanted to lose body fat, she thought she needed to eat less food a day, when actually she needed to eat *more* nutrient-rich food that served her.

Let's take a closer look at Justine's food log for one day:

Sample Food Log	Prot (g)	Fat (g)	Sat (g)	Carbs (g)	Sugar (g)	Fibre (g)	Cals (kcal)
Breakfast							
Protein Shake 1 scoop (35g)	26	2.5	1	3	2	1	140
What is the sweetener in this shake?							
Frozen Mixed Berries 1 cup	1	0	0	17	11	3	70
Skim of Nonfat Milk (Calcium Fortified) 1 cup	8.4	0.44	0.289	11.98	11.98	0	86
A lot of sugar to start your day with.							
Total	35.4	2.94	1.289	31.98	24.98	4	296
Lunch ? Could you add vegetables to lunch to increase fibre and micronutrients?							
Skinless Chicken Breast 1/2 breast, bone and skin removed	27.25	1.46	0.389	0	0	0	130
Dinner							
Snacks/Other				There is a lot of sugar in grapes.			
Grapes (Red or Green) European Type Varieties such as Thompson Seedless) 1 cup, seedless	1.15	0.26	0.086	28.96	24.77	1.4	110
Protein Bar 1 bar (60g)	21	8	3	21	1	17	210
Total	22.15	8.26	very low	49.96	25.77 enough? ?	18.4	320
Total	84.8	12.66	4.764	81.94	50.75	22.4	746

more moderate   OK   high !   very low

As you can see, Justine did not eat dinner that day. Skipping meals would be fine if Justine ate enough nutrient-rich food throughout the day. Upon reflection, Justine recalled that she hadn't eaten because she was too busy driving her kids to their sports practices that evening. The problem was that Justine's energy was low, her sleep was inadequate, she was moody, her body composition lacked muscle tone and her sex drive was low. As well, she found herself losing her patience with her kids and husband, and her menstrual cycles were severe. Justine hoped that a change in her nutrition would help her to feel better.

Justine's ASSESSment from Three Days of TRACKing:

What three things are you learning from tracking your food and water intake? Number one is that not being prepared leads to making poor food choices that are only quick fixes. The second is that there is a lot of sugar and vegetable oil in products I have been eating. The third thing I've learned is that I am on top of my water consumption, and my protein intake is fairly consistent.

Can you see any patterns? If yes, explain. I have noticed that when I preplan my meals I am more likely to grocery shop accordingly, and when I am not prepared, I grab whatever is on hand with limited good choices to choose from.

Do you see room for improvement? Explain (either way). Absolutely! I need to meal-plan and have food readily available in my home that I can eat. I need to get better at organizing the busy days/nights in our home, and start using my crockpot or meal prep earlier in the week. I need to find snack options that have less sugar in them. I have always been a snacker and need to ensure that these snacks do not sabotage progress I am making.

What you are doing well that you want to continue? I would like to continue to consume my water throughout the day (I always have my water bottle with me). I would like to continue to raise my awareness of the food I am eating. I have had sensitivities to wheat in particular since childhood and know that I feel better when it is limited in my diet. I am open to trying new foods, searching out grain-free recipes, and have found some favourites but will continue to find new options.

Justine's Answers to ASSESSment Questions
(Scale of 1 to 10 with 1 = poor; 10 = excellent).

1. How is your digestion? Why? My digestion is a six. I had an upset stomach one day last week, but for the most part it has been decent. I had a little gas and bloating. I believe that stress impacts my digestion as well as how I eat (both obviously need to improve).

2. How is your sleep? Why? I'd give my sleep a seven. At times I find I have trouble turning my brain off at night.

The day's events (as well as the days to come) run through my mind. I often think there are not enough hours in the day or days in the week. I need to better prioritize what needs to be done.

3. How is your mood? Why? My mood is a seven on the scale. I am often short with others, or easily disappointed when they haven't lived up to my expectations (which I assumed they would just know). We are in a transition period, with family living with us right now; [so many] people under one roof can be stressful as we try to manage everyone's schedules. While somewhat overwhelmed with finding appropriate substitutes, I am optimistic about the changes I am making,

4. How is your energy? Why? I'm a seven. I often wake up tired in the morning and feel exhausted in the afternoons and evenings.

Justine knows these things because she TRACKed and then ASSESSed. Next, Justine can begin to ADJUST, based on what she learns about nutrition in the NOURISH lessons.

What About You?

After three days of TRACKing, you can start to delve into what your food logs mean. It is time to ASSESS. Now you can begin to take charge of your nutrition so that you are flooding your cells with just the right amount of nutrient-rich food, every day, specifically for you. It's time to discover your own nutritional tipping points using your digestion, sleep, mood and energy levels as your compass.

View your food log summary on your nutrition tracking app. Plan to do this weekly, every Sunday night, throughout the program.

List three things you are learning from TRACKing your food and water intake. Can you see any patterns? If yes, explain. Do you see room for improvement? Explain (either way):

Make a list of what you are already doing well that you want to continue.

Now, ask the four ASSESSment questions. Number your answers on a scale of 1 to 10 (1 = poor; 10 = excellent):

How is you digestion? Why?

How is your sleep? Why?

How is your mood? Why?

How is your energy level? Why?

You are learning what I discovered from working with hundreds of clients, people like you, over the last 10+ years. If there is one thing I understand about food it is this: **Food is personal.** It stimulates an emotional response in us, and it rules all. Feed yourself poorly, and you will find it difficult to be at the top of your game in any aspect of your life! Something will always be "off." NOURISH is pretty simple: **figure out how to feed yourself, and everything gets better.** Vanity aside—even health aside—when you get the right, nutrient-rich food you need into your cells, your gut and your brain get better, and therefore, so do you. It's that simple.

Here are some other thoughts from NOURISH clients about TRACKing their food:

Make food logging the number one priority—do not procrastinate! It's there to guide you. The lesson I am learning is that I need to preplan my food for more than a day or two.

—Trina, NOURISH client

I had lots of big aha moments during the first week of tracking. One of them was when I realized how completely ignorant I was when it came to food. I started to learn about what is healthy and what pretends to be healthy. The nutrients—or lack thereof—don't lie.

—Dinah, NOURISH client

READER'S NOTES:

PART II: NOURISH

CHAPTER ELEVEN

What is right is forsaken for what is convenient.
–Johann Wolfgang van Goethe

A Calorie Is Not A Calorie.

A calorie is not a calorie? What does this mean? Let's say you decide to follow a traditional diet that is 2000 calories for a man and 1200 calories for a woman. What foods make up the calories for the day? Fast food? What if you eat only vegetables and no protein? What about eating only cake and ice cream?

Remember what I said about being overfed and under NOURISHed? If you are over-fat or if you are losing lean muscle mass because you are unintentionally starving yourself, your body could store fat from every calorie you consume, whether it comes from healthy food or not.

For example, people who do not eat enough calories daily from protein or healthy fats daily can sometimes end up what is often referred to as "skinny-fat." They look lean but carry a spare tire of fat around their midsections. Skinny-fat refers to the fact that muscle weighs more than fat and people who are not feeding their muscle on a regular basis could be losing muscle and storing fat. This is what makes them lighter on the scale. This is what happens to some people when they diet by cutting calories without paying attention to their nutrient needs. Dieters who focus on calories, but do not focus on nutrient rich foods, may become lighter on the scale. The lower number on the scale pleases dieters initially. But, over time, people who consume a low calorie, nutrient deficient diet may find that their energy is depleted, their skin looks grey and sags and their faces look drawn and gaunt. Once the euphoria of seeing a smaller number on the scale wanes, there isn't much left to celebrate.

On NOURISH, you will focus on consuming nutrient rich foods that feed every cell in your body. Feeding your cells helps you to release excess body fat, or if you are too lean, gain body fat. NOURISHing yourself with enough calories of the right nutrient rich foods (for you) will help you to maintain your lean muscle mass as you age and, possibly, help you to gain more lean muscle mass. This is a very good thing as lean muscle helps to keep your metabolism humming!

Let's figure out the minimum number of calories you need per day based on your age, your lean mass (as per your metric body fat measurements from the **Your Starting Point** chapter), and your actual weight on the scale.

Basal Metabolic Rate (BMR)—What Is Yours?

The Basal Metabolic Rate (BMR) is the baseline number of calories you need daily to stay alive and kicking. I am not talking about working, playing, exercising and enduring any kind of stress—good or bad!

I mean consuming enough calories so that you do not start eating yourself from the inside out and wasting away. The medical term for wasting like this is catabolizing[8]. Even if you are overly fat, catabolization of healthy body tissues is something you do not want to have happen. People who do not consume enough nutrient-rich calories in a day end up losing lean muscle mass. Catabolization, in otherwise healthy people, can show up like this:

A person can be over fat and therefore storing fat by holding onto every single calorie consumed from nutrient-dead, fast food because the body is *starving* for nutrients. This can be true even if the food has been deemed healthy by North American society's standards.

A person can be under-fat due to consumption of too few calories. Even if the calories come from healthy sources—again, the body is starving.

Some of the results for people who do not consume enough nutrient-rich food depend on genetics. We may have a tendency towards either being lean or carrying extra body fat. However, for many people, as I stated at the start of NOURISH, body composition is determined by stress and lifestyle. Life is about managing stress proactively—not reactively. It is important to note that the body does not discriminate between good stress and bad stress. Job changes are stressful, falling in love is stressful, moving triggers stress, death and dying around you cause obvious stress. Even good sex is stressful!

You might be shocked to learn that my leanest clients eat the most calories on a daily basis, but it's true. I work with healthy, fit women who are 10 per cent body fat who eat 2000+ calories per day. And I work with healthy, fit men who are five per cent body fat, who eat 3000+ calories per day.

Conversely, I have female clients who are 25 per cent+ body fat, who eat under 1000 calories per day, as well as men who are 18 per cent+ body fat, who eat under 1500 calories per day. Often, these people try to work out more to counteract their higher body fat percentages. This backfires on them, and they end up storing even more body fat. And, sometimes, the over exercising causes them to *lose* lean muscle mass!

My heaviest clients, the people with a high ratio of body fat to lean muscle mass—even if they are light on the scale (skinny-fat)—are often the ones who eat the least. This is because fat weighs less than muscle. But, as you may already know, fat takes up more room than muscle. That is why I can weigh 145 pounds and wear a size six and another woman who is my height and build can weigh 145 and wear a size 12.

Think about that for a minute...

I always make sure that what I am "seeing" lines up with the results from client's metrics and food logs. For example, I have female clients who are 10 per cent body fat, and male clients who are five per cent body fat, who are unhealthy. These people lack muscle tone, their skin is dry and often itchy (possibly due to eating a very low-fat diet), their energy is low, and their immune systems are down. Many of these people (who could be referred to as skinny-fat) are sick all year long; they catch every bug that comes down the pike. And their families are sick, too. In my research, our bodies are a reflection of their food logs and lifestyle choices.

Calories: BMR versus Body Mass Index (BMI)

Do not confuse your Basal Metabolic Rate (BMR) with the standard doctor's office Body Mass Index (BMI) measurement. They are not the same. The issue with the BMI is that it does not account for lean mass (muscle, bones, blood, body water, organs, etc.), activity level, or diet. Someone who is fit and muscular may have a BMI that would be considered high to unhealthy, but they might be only 10 per cent body fat. As a mesomorph body type*, I am like that:

I am 5'5" and 145 pounds.

I have about 13 pounds of body fat and 132 pounds of lean mass.

I am 10 per cent body fat and a true mesomorph body type. Which for me means that if I get fat, I get fat everywhere; if I lean out, I lean out everywhere.

If I weighed what the BMI says I should, I would be under-fat, would look drawn, and potentially be sick all the time. Weighing 125 pounds would not work for my frame and muscle mass—I would look malnourished!

Understanding your body fat percentage and where you fit on the body fat metrics table is a healthier and more educated way to manage your health and wellness. Plus, always consider how you feel. How is your digestion? How is your sleep and your mood and your energy level? Remember in the **Your Starting Point** chapter how many ways the scale can lie? The BMI is not a reliable tool to measure your health.

*Do you want to know your body type? Take an online quiz:
http://www.bodybuilding.com/fun/becker3.htm
http://www.youthink.com/quiz.cfm

http://www.proprofs.com/quiz-school/story.php?title=what-is-your-body-type_1

How To Calculate Your BMR

For NOURISH, you will use your specific BMR calories per day as your baseline for how much nutrient-rich food to consume per day. Again, this is not a perfect science. We are using these calculations as a place to springboard from on your journey to wellness. And, these numbers mean nothing unless your TRACK, ASSESS and ADJUST based on your findings.

To find your BMR, go back to the **Your Starting Point** chapter and review your body fat measurements and plug them in below:

Your Body Fat Per Cent: _____
Your Body Fat: _____ lb.
Your Lean Body Mass: _____ lb.

Next, Use The Katch-McArdle Equation To Calculate Your BMR.

Multiple your lean body mass pounds number (see above) by 9.79759519
Then add 370.
The resulting number is your BMR.
Record your BMR here:_____

The equation above provides an estimate for the minimum amount of calories to shoot for daily. Here are the general guides that I use for my clients for daily caloric minimums:

Women:
smaller framed: BMR @ 1200–1400
medium framed: BMR @ 1500–1700
larger framed: BMR @ 1800–2000+
Men:
smaller framed: BMR @ 1800–2100
medium framed: BMR @ 2200–2500
larger framed: BMR @ 2600–3000+

Total Daily Energy Expenditure (TDEE): What is Yours?

Now, let's account for real life. Remember I said that your BMR helps to estimate your minimum amount of daily calories required just to stay alive? Your Total Daily Energy Expenditure (TDEE) is the number of calories you need to consume daily if you are doing anything other than lounging around all day[9]. This would include things like work, raising kids, household chores, hobbies, exercise, sex, and, all other forms of daily stress—both positive (taking a trip) and negative (a death in the family).

Your TDEE is determined by considering your actual body weight on the scale, your lean body mass (calculated from your body fat metrics and recorded in the **Your Starting Point** chapter), your daily activity level (see below), and your age. To calculate your TDEE, multiply your BMR by your activity factor.

1.1–1.2 = Sedentary (desk job, and little formal exercise)

1.3–1.4 = Lightly Active (light daily activity and light exercise 1–3 days a week)

1.5–1.6 = Moderately Active (moderate daily activity and moderate exercise 3–5 days a week)

1.7–1.8 = Very Active (physically demanding lifestyle and hard exercise 6–7 days a week)

1.9–2.2 = Extremely Active (athletes in endurance training or those with very hard physical jobs)[10]

For my clients, I generally use 1.5 for their calculations. This allows us to stay in a conservative range if the goal is to lose body fat and gain lean mass. It is a good choice for beginners because most people greatly over-estimate how hard they actually exercise. Remember, these calculations are estimates to give you a range to aim for daily. They are only useful combined with the TAAP system and the nutrition lessons you are about to learn on the NOURISH program. Recall the title of this chapter: **A Calorie is Not a Calorie**.

Let's Look At My BMR And TDEE:

Step One: Calculate BMR

My lean mass is 133 lb. x 9.79759519 + 370 = 1673 calories per day. My BMR = 1673 calories per day.

Step Two: Calculate TDEE

1673 (BMR) x 1.5 = 2593 calories per day. My TDEE is anywhere between 2000 and 2500 calories per day to maintain the lean mass I have and to keep my body fat in a range that works for me.

MY TDEE = 2000–2500 calories per day

If you who have been consuming very low numbers of calories for years and you do not work out regularly, I recommend staying between the BMR and the *bottom* end of the TDEE. For me, that would mean between 1673 and 2000 calories per day. The 1673 calories per day (my BMR) helps to ensure that I do not lose lean muscle mass by sliding into starvation mode. The 2000+ range allows me to work out, maintain my lean muscle mass as I age, and have enough energy for day-to-day life. If you have non-essential body fat to lose, staying between the BMR and the bottom end of the TDEE is helpful. If you need to *gain* body fat, add an additional 300 to 500 calories to your TDEE.

These are the basic guidelines I use for TDEE ranges for my clients:

Women: (moderately active)

smaller framed: TDEE @ 1400–1600+

medium framed: TDEE @ 1600–2000+

larger framed: TDEE @ 2000–2500+

Men: (moderately active)

smaller framed: TDEE @ 2000–2400+

medium framed: TDEE @ 2500–2900+

larger framed: TDEE @ 2600–3000++

ASSESS Your Food Logs. What do they mean?

First, how many calories are you consuming?

      Write down your highest calorie day:

      Write down your lowest calorie day:

      Write down your daily average for three days:

Don't panic! NOURISH is not about counting calories. However, you do need to know whether you are meeting your caloric minimums. Are you eating enough nutrient-rich calories to do what you want every day? How is your digestion, your sleep, your mood and your energy level?

I still have some days when I am not eating enough! I cannot believe how much food I can actually eat on this program. It is challenging to change my mindset after so many years of eating "like a lady should." But, I can feel the difference when I do.

                                  –Abigail, NOURISH client

Again, ask: What am I hungry for? And, What am I getting for what I am eating?

Figure out where your caloric range is and stay in it. And, stay curious. Caloric ranges are subject to change as life changes. For example, if after six weeks on NOURISH, you start working out, you may require more calories. If you change from an active job to a desk job, you may need to ADJUST your caloric intake.

Believe it or not, on NOURISH it is better to go *over* your caloric range than *under*. A common theme I see when coaching clients and reviewing their initial food logs is that most people do not eat enough calories. Start to use your BMR and TDEE caloric amounts to organize your daily nutrient intake. If you tend to eat low calorie and you don't plan ahead, at bedtime you might be 500 calories shy of your minimum. (My client Justine discovered this after she TRACKed her food the first week.) Instead, preplan your meals the day before, enter them into your nutrient tracker and see what your total calories are for the next day. Even better is to plan out your entire week of meals. Also, don't "save" calories so you can eat junk food. Just go over your calories and start fresh with the next meal. If you skip meals and therefore, nutrients, to have cake, you will be starving yourself! Know that it is fine for your meal plan to be subject to change as your nutrition knowledge increases on the NOURISH program.

Next, we look at macronutrients: protein, fats, and carbohydrates. Macronutrients are essential for optimal health and are only available from our food sources. This is why it is so important to eat nutrient rich, whole foods that serve us!

CHAPTER TWELVE

Facts do not cease to exist because they are ignored.
—Aldous Huxley

The Macronutrients: Protein

Protein is a major building block for our bodies that helps us to build and maintain lean muscle mass, satiates us, and fuels us. According to the Institute of Medicine, we should get at least 10 per cent of our daily calories, but not more than 35 per cent, from protein. You need to remember this: eat your protein minimums every day. This means a minimum of 56 grams for men and 46 grams for women.[11]

Eating your protein minimums daily is one of the most important aspects of NOURISH. Meeting our protein grams minimums daily prevents what is called protein turn-over,[12] so our bodies don't "turn-in" on themselves (remember catabolization?). You might even eat up to one gram of protein per pound of your lean body mass (for example: I might eat 130+ grams of protein per day). Consider this if you are an athlete and you train hard. Hard could equal several hours per day or 10+ hours per week. In my research, most of my clients do well with a moderate approach to protein. I have found that women do well between 60 to 100 grams per day (more if they are elite athletes) and men do well between 100 and 150 grams per day (again, more if they are elite athletes). Regardless, you need to meet your minimums of protein grams every day.

Too Much Protein?

In the nutrition world, there is a belief that too much protein can be stored as fat. If you are someone who stores fat easily or who is not exercising, shoot for a moderate approach to your protein intake but eat at least your minimum grams per

day. **Warning: regardless of your body composition, do
not fall into the trap of just eating protein all day long.**
Eating too much protein could leave you too full for the two
other macronutrients, healthy fats and carbohydrates and fibre.

How much protein you may require daily can depend
many factors including age, lifestyle and genetics. For example, a 6'5", lean, 185-pound, male, office worker who does
not work out is not going to need as much as his 230-pound,
twin who is a professional football player. A woman in her
childbearing years may utilize more protein than her grandmother. A high-powered, fit, lawyer working an 80-hour
workweek may have the same protein needs as a steel
worker—both are stressful careers.

I ask all my clients to make sure they are eating their
minimums—for both calories and protein—especially if they
have been in a deficit. You can't know how many grams of
protein you are consuming daily unless you TRACK. This is
part of what the first three days of TRACKing on NOURISH
was all about. Usually, when people start NOURISH they
have no idea about how much protein they consume in a day.
You may not either unless you TRACK! Get your protein
grams to at least your minimum grams per day. Again, my
research has shown that men benefit from between 100 to
150 grams of protein per day and many women do well on
between 60 to 100 grams of protein per day. (Note: elite athletes may require more protein daily.) No matter what, make
sure you eat your minimum requirement for protein per day:
for men that means 56 grams and for women it's 46 grams.

Healthy Protein Sources for NOURISH (organic if possible):

- grass-fed only meats
- wild-caught fish
- raw nuts
- grass-fed only whey protein supplements

Remember, I asked you to TRACK three days of your regular feedings, so you could ASSESS your trends. You need to see where you started, so you can begin to ADJUST, so you can make PROGRESS. If you have been feeling low in energy, you lack muscle tone, and you are hungry all the time, maybe it is because you have not been eating enough protein daily. Start to proactively plan your protein feedings into your meals. I suggest you begin to cook in bulk once or twice per week, so you always have healthy protein options available to you. Another idea is to hard boil a dozen eggs and stock your refrigerator with full fat cheeses and yogurts. Beware of quick and easy, processed protein choices like convenience store jerky. Many store bought beef jerkies are full of artificial fla- vourings that are counterproductive to eating real, unproc- essed foods that serve you. *(Always read the labels of any packaged foods before you purchase any food item.)* If there is something on the label that you cannot pronounce, put it back and make a healthier choice. Also, beware of "natural flavourings." If the flavourings are natural, ask yourself why the company won't list them?

A Note About Soy

If possible (and it is always possible), avoid soy and soy prod- ucts. Soy is a phytoestrogen (a plant estrogen) that can wreak havoc on our hormones. Soy can cause digestive issues, lower immune system function, affect memory and fertility. Many other ailments like food allergies, kidney stones, breast cancer and heart disease now include soy as a culprit.[13]

A Note About Protein Shakes

Should you use protein shakes? Sure. Shakes are convenient, are a great source of protein, and offer another way to in- crease your water intake. Don't hesitate to shop around and try different types of protein shakes to find the one that works best for you. Read the labels. Make sure your protein shake is:

- free of artificial sweeteners. (No Splenda either—also called sucralose. See list of names for sugar in the **Game Changer Number Two: S-U-G-A-R** chapter.)
- fructose free (yes, that's right—no fruit sugars).
- two carbs or less.
- fibre-less or does not have chicory root or inulin as a fibre source.
- whey, or pea, or rice protein based (whey is the first choice).
- not containing any stimulants.

Also, make sure your shake is palatable! If you have to hold your nose to drink it, then something is wrong. Try another brand.

Note: Do not over-blend your protein powders. You want the protein to break down in the body, not in the blender. Add your powder last, and just pulse it a bit or use a shaker bottle.

A Note About Vegetarianism

I was a vegetarian for about 10 years. As an animal lover, I started in my early teens for ethical reasons. I then cited political and environmental reasons for being vegetarian. After a while, I realized that I was a vegetarian out of habit and because I thought it might make me leaner. In my experience, the NOURISH program is hard to follow if you are a vegetarian. I do not know how you can keep your carbohydrates and sugars at reasonable levels living on grains and legumes and I do not recommend soy products of any kind. I don't believe that you can live on pasta and tofu and stay healthy. NOURISH is not a program for vegetarians.

Look Back at Your Food Logs

Remember, we truly are what we eat. Do not buy cheap protein unless you want a less-than-optimal body.

> How many grams of protein are you averaging per day?
>
> What was your highest protein day
>
> What was your lowest protein day?
>
> Did you meet the minimum grams of protein per day?

TAAP: TRACK, ASSESS and ADJUST, to PROGRESS

Recall Dr. Freedhoff's quote from the start of NOURISH: "Fear the nutrition guru whose opinions don't change." As you learn more, be open to what works for your body and what does not. Along with TRACKing, it is important to continually ASSESS how you feel so that you can make ADJUSTments to your nutrition in order to make PROGRESS. You are in the process of discovering your nutritional tipping points.

Now, let's look at the next macronutrient. Let's take a look at healthy fats.

CHAPTER THIRTEEN

It is a narrow mind which cannot look at a subject from various points of view.
—George Eliot

The Macronutrients: Fats

First, and this is very important: **healthy fat does not make you fat!** The dieting industry has sabotaged our eating habits over the last 30 years with misinformation about dietary fats. We can credit Ancel Keys for that. Keys was an epidemiologist who hypothesized that dietary fat was the cause of heart disease.[14] And because grains are cheaper and easier to store than fats and protein, grains have become the cheap and easy way to feed the world. Here is a question: Why is it that with the fat-free, high carbohydrate diets of the last several decades society has gotten fatter and fatter, and heart disease, brain diseases (like dementia and Alzheimer's) and diabetes have gone through the roof? One answer is because *we need fat.* Fat is an essential macronutrient!

Moving forward, consume full-fat dairy (preferably organic) and animal proteins (preferably free-range) to increase your healthy fat profile. Eat fat from plant and animal sources daily. Say YES to whole milk, yogurt, and cheeses. Say YES to butter! Say YES to heavy cream in your coffee (use cream and you won't miss sugar). Say YES to red meat once or twice a week. Say YES to higher calorie nuts like cashews and Macadamia. And, say Yes to avocados!

We need fat to feel satisfied. We need fat for our brains.

Essential fatty acids and cholesterol are key to all of the cells in the body. And, healthy fats power our metabolism.[15] Healthy fats help to regulate our hormones, and especially as we age—hormones rule! Hormones are chemical messengers that help to regulate all of our bodily functions including everything from thirst to sex drive. Our brains and our guts rule our hormones and we need them to work together for our bodies to be balanced. Insulin is the hormone that tells the body to store fat. The hormone Leptin manages the amount of Insulin we have in our bodies. Leptin is also known as the satiety hormone and affects all of the hormones in the body. If either hormone, Insulin or Leptin, is out of balance then, potentially, so are we![16]

Something is wrong with our current, culturally acceptable, low-fat, no-fat diets; it's showing up everywhere. Think about all of the fat-phobic people who eat extremely low fat and have for years! If you have been living on a low-calorie and low-fat diet:

> Are you carrying too much body fat?
> Is your cholesterol through the roof?
> Is your blood sugar uncontrollable?
> Are you moody, emotional, cranky, or angry?
> Are you hungry all the time, even if you are eating all the time?

Are you ever so hungry and shaky that you get mad? That's the "hangries" coming out, because you are a sugar burner instead of a fat burner. Good news! Eating healthy fats, every day, will help to satiate you so you won't feel hungry all the time; you will, in fact, be more NOURISHed. If you are someone who snacks all day long, you may find that when you up your healthy fat intake, you no longer need to graze all day long.

And the bonus is that when you eat fat, you will burn fat.

I realized that I was finally able to hear what my body was telling me…that it craved, savoured, and thrived on plenty of healthy fats!
—Trina, NOURISH client

Sources of Healthy Fats (organic if possible):

- olives and olive oil
- coconut oil and unsweetened coconut
- raw nuts and nut butters (almonds, walnuts, cashews, macadamia, pecans, pistachios, Brazil nuts)
- grass-fed meats (beef, chicken, pork, lamb, venison, bison)
- wild caught salmon (Do not eat farmed fish. Read labels carefully!)
- whole milk dairy products (cheeses, heavy cream, yogurts, kefir)
- whole milk goat products (cheeses, milks and yogurts)
- organic eggs from pasture raised chickens
- palm oil
- butter (preferably organic)
- unheated, organic walnut oil
- avocados and avocado oil

Note: Do not use olive oil for high heat cooking, as it turns rancid. Coconut oil and butter are the best fats for high heat cooking.[17] If you don't like the taste of coconut, look for unscented coconut oil options at the health food store or online.

When asked what she wished she had done sooner on the NOURISH program, Jessica said, "Eat avocados—something so simple with so many benefits. I have less muscle soreness after workouts, which I'm attributing to the changes I have made—especially adding in more fats and drinking my water."

Gradually Increase Your Healthy Fats Daily

Look back at your first food log. If you have been eating below 50 per cent fat per day of your total calories, make sure to increase your daily dose of healthy fats *slowly*. For example, if you have been eating 20 grams of fat per day, do not suddenly increase your fats to over 100 grams per day. Any change in your diet—even if it is healthy—can be stressful on the body. Always give your body time to adjust.

The easiest way to start incorporating healthy fats into your diet is to make the switch from non-fat and light dairy to full fat. The next time you are at the grocery store, compare the labels of a non-fat yogurt to a whole milk yogurt. Fat brings flavour and texture to our foods making them more palatable. When the food industry took fat out of our foods, they had to put in additives and fillers (like extra sugar) to make products taste better.

You can put healthy fats in your protein shakes, you can add good oils (see lists) to salads in the form of homemade dressings, and you can snack on nuts—even higher calorie nuts like cashews and macadamia! Try avocados plain, with horseradish, or just salt them and eat them with a spoon. Add avocados to your shakes and salads. Many people shy away from avocados because of their high (healthy) fat content and high calories. On NOURISH, you can eat avocados guilt-free. Learn to love avocados if you don't already. To up your healthy fats, you can also put butter on your veggies. Butter helps the body to assimilate the minerals and fat-soluble nutrients in vegetables, so they can be better used in the body.[18]

How to Gradually Increase Your Healthy Fats:
You could carry nuts in your purse or bag for snacks on the road. And, you can make up a dozen hard-boiled eggs for the fridge every week. For a snack, eat a tablespoon of almond butter. Cook with coconut oil and put some in your tea or coffee or, eat a tablespoon straight—just like nut butters. And, of course, you can cook with butter.

Note: Refrigerate your fats so they have a longer shelf life (except for coconut oil—it turns solid when cold). Rancid oils and nuts not only taste bad, they are not healthy.

By adding in more fats, I noticed a change in what I was craving. I don't want to eat chips, candy, and chocolate because my body is getting what it needs. I eat REAL food and limit processed foods. It is a little more challenging and can be more expensive than the junky processed foods, BUT I feel I am absolutely worth it.

–Justine, NOURISH client

Do Not Consume Vegetable Oils

Did you notice that canola, grape seed and all other so-called healthy vegetable oils were not on the list of healthy fats? Vegetable oils are highly processed and are prone to rancidity. Vegetable oils can damage DNA, which could cause cancer. They can contribute to building arterial plaques associated with cardiovascular disease. And, vegetable oils also contribute to premature aging, wrinkles and inflammation[19] (like headaches, gut aches, and joint aches). **This means that you need to make your own dressings and sauces.** Store bought dressings and sauces are full of bad oils and sugar!

What About Trans Fats?

Processed trans fats are detrimental to our health. Trans fats can be found in non-nutritive sources like packaged foods, fried foods and margarine. The body does not recognize trans fats as real food.[20] Stay away from them. If the food you are about to eat won't rot, avoid it at all costs.

Moving Forward...

Always ask, What am I hungry for? And, ask What am I getting for what I am eating? Make sure to read every label on everything you eat and assume that restaurants (and your family and friends) are using unhealthy vegetable oils, unless you ask. Remember, for high heat cooking, use butter or coconut oil. Olive oil goes rancid at high heat. Use olive oil for low heat cooking and for salad dressings.

Once again, do not fear healthy fats. Fat will not make you fat. Eat healthy fats to burn fat.

All the information out there about what to eat is so confusing. They tell you not to eat fat, not to eat eggs, to eat whole grains, etc. NOURISH taught me not to be afraid of fat. Now, I pay attention to using the right types of fat. Fat-free and low fat, doesn't serve me anymore. I make sure I have coconut oil, avocados, and nuts on a regular basis. If I eat yogurt, I add a few tablespoons of flax and hemp seeds with it, and I just buy the plain, full fat, Greek style instead of the fruity ones.

—Avery, NOURISH client

Understanding that eating fat will help you to burn fat is one of the most challenging mental hurdles of NOURISH. This is especially true if you have been eating a traditional low-fat, high carbohydrate, low-calorie diet. But if what you have been doing has not worked, or it only works for a while and then backfires—what have you got to lose? Maybe it is time to try something else. Up your healthy fats slowly and eat fats from a variety of sources. For example, don't just eat nuts and olive oil. And, don't consume more than one avocado per day. Try walnut oil on your salads, make some guacamole dip for your veggies and try some new cheeses.

> How many grams of fat did you consume on average?
> Lightest day? (amount and day of the week)
> Highest day? (amount and day of the week)

Many of my clients find that when they gradually increase their healthy fats, they notice a marked improvement in digestion, sleep, mood, skin, and cravings (this is one is huge).

Experiment, be curious, ASSESS and ADJUST. Using the TAAP system, you will find your nutritional tipping point for your daily dose of healthy fats. Consider the old saying that *you are what you eat.* If you eat cheap and easy, non-nutritive food, again you will have a less than optimal body and mind. Remember your NOURISH compasses to find your nutritional tipping points? Check in and ask: how is your sleep, digestion, mood and energy level? And ask, *What am I getting for what I am eating?*

I realize that this chapter on fats can be a lot to take in. My advice is to reread the whole chapter. As a matter of fact, re-read all of the macronutrient chapters, multiple times. Sometimes we get information turned around in our minds unless we revisit it again and again until we've got it. Remember, on the NOURISH program, you are looking to find your own nutritional tipping points. As you make changes with your nutrition, your body will change. Stay curious and revisit the lessons often.

Next, we move onto the third macronutrient, carbohydrates.

CHAPTER FOURTEEN

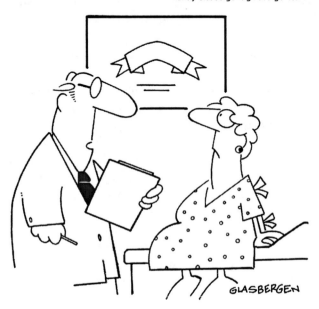

© Randy Glasbergen / glasbergen.com

"The high-carb diet I put you on 20 years ago gave you diabetes, high blood pressure and heart disease. Oops."

The Macronutrients: Carbohydrates

The third macronutrient is carbohydrate. Carbohydrates provide an immediate source of energy for the body's cells. We need carbs for the body to function properly. Here is the most important concept for you to grasp: **Your body does not discriminate amongst carbohydrates.** The complex carbohydrate of vegetables and grain, and the simple sugars in fruits and candy, all register as sugar in the body.

Carbohydrates are split into two groups: simple and complex. Simple carbohydrates (mono and disaccharides) can be found in processed foods. Complex carbohydrates (polysac-charides) are found in whole foods, like vegetables and grains. The difference between simple and complex is that simple carbs are digested much faster than complex carbs.[21]

We begin to produce Insulin (the fat-storing hormone) as soon as we think about eating. This is also true when we anticipate eating our favourite carbohydrate-dense foods and sweets.[22] Think about that the next time you have a craving for potato chips, or want to pick up a chocolate bar at the grocery store check out or you see a late night commercial for pizza!

Contrary to what you might think, the NOURISH program is not down on carbohydrates. But poor and plentiful carbohydrates from low or non-nutritive sources are making us fat, anxious, sleepless and full of digestive issues. NOURISH is about teaching yourself through TAAP to make smart carbohydrate choices for a better digestion, sleep, mood, and energy levels. And, smart carbs help us to acquire or maintain a healthier body composition. Again, NOURISH is not a low-carb diet. NOURISH promotes a smart carb lifestyle. With NOURISH, I'm asking you to continually ask, *What am I getting for what I am eating?* I am asking you to think about your carbohydrate sources on this program. You want to learn to make smart carb choices for y-o-u. The takeaway for you in this chapter is: *Carbs are not the enemy but all carbs are not created equal!*

Healthy Sources of Carbohydrates:

- vegetables
- nuts and seeds
- avocados
- coconut (unsweetened)
- berries
- lemons
- limes

What challenged me most about NOURISH? Vegetables. I am not a veggie eater. But I am now on speaking terms with broccoli and cauliflower. And olives! [I] never knew they tasted so good.

–Bill, NOURISH client

Low-Carbohydrate Vegetables:

- arugula
- cucumbers
- broccoli raab
- celery
- white mushrooms
- radishes
- turnips
- romaine lettuce
- asparagus
- green pepper
- okra
- cauliflower
- green, red and yellow peppers
- cabbage
- broccoli
- spinach
- green beans
- kale
- sugar snap peas
- onions

It is time to get over any hang-ups you may have about eating enough calories, and consuming healthy fats. And, it is time to eat more vegetables! When you embrace the concepts of NOURISH, you will begin to burn fat instead of sugar. And that is when the real changes in your body chemistry and your body composition will start to occur. What could this mean? You could release non-essential body fat, you could gain more lean muscle mass and you could experience fewer mood swings. Your quality of sleep might improve and your need to eat every couple of hours might diminish. A higher sex drive, a calmer, more focused mind, and more energy are all possible too! And, you could see improvement in your blood chemistry profile. It's important to check in with your doctor regularly to monitor your progress.

Questions:

How many grams of carbohydrates did you consume on average?
Lightest day? (amount and day of the week)
Highest day? (amount and day of the week)

Look back at your carbohydrate numbers...

If you were over 200 grams per day, shoot for less than 200 grams.
If you were less than 200 grams, shoot for around 150 grams.
If you were less than 150 grams, shoot for around 100 grams.
If you were less than 100 grams, shoot for not lower than 50 grams per day.

To be clear, some very low carb diets advocate consuming less than 50 grams per day of carbohydrate, and part of some programs prescribe less than 30 grams per day. In my experience, eating a diet this low in carbohydrates is not sustainable. Beyond bad breath and brain fog, I've also found that anything lower than 50 grams per day makes working out at high intensities very, very tough. As I mentioned, I find that once clients start to cut back on nutrient-dead carbs and sugar (and they eat adequate protein and up their healthy fats), they have less cravings.

Do not make the mistake of eating too low carbohydrate, on a continual basis, to speed up fat loss. Again, in my experience, this is not sustainable and doing so will cause rapid weight gain the moment you get your carbs back into even moderate levels. Do not be afraid of healthy carbs as long as they are smart carb choices that are higher in fibre and low in sugar. We will discuss how to do this more extensively in **The Game Changer** chapters on fibre and sugar.

Optimal Grams of Carbohydrate

To determine your optimal grams of carbohydrate per day, ask yourself what you are getting from the number of grams and the quality of the carbs you are eating? It is time to ask the four ASSESSment questions to find your nutritional tipping point for carbs. How is your digestion? How is your sleep? How is your mood? How is your energy level?

For me, my optimal range is between 80 and 100 grams of nutrient-rich carbohydrates per day. Not 45 grams and not 150 grams. I discovered this by experimenting using the TAAP system. I could not have known where my tipping point was until I TRACKed, ASSESSed, and ADJUSTed. I kept checking in with my digestion, my sleep, my mood and my energy levels as my compass. From there, I was able to make educated decisions about my choices and PROGRESS. If I eat too many carbs, I feel sluggish and bloated and my monkey mind goes into overdrive. For example, this happens for me if I eat something like too many blueberries at one time! I am better off to have a half-cup of berries versus a whole cup to cut back on the sugar. Conversely, if my carbs get too low, I can't sleep and I cannot work out at a high intensity level. I get something I call "carb drag." And, carb drag is a total drag!

If you have been eating a carbohydrate-heavy diet, say 200+ grams per day, when you start to wean your carb grams down, you might go through a bit of a detox period. Signs of detoxing might include things like headaches or crankiness and cravings. You might experience digestive changes including possible diarrhea, constipation, gas and bloating and increased or decreased trips to the bathroom (make sure to drink your water!)

Do not worry! TAAP, drink your water daily and keep your focus on eating adequate, high quality protein, healthy fats and fibre rich, low sugar, smart carb choices. As you find your nutritional tipping point with your carbs, it's the water, the protein, and the healthy fats that will ease your cravings and help to level off your digestion, sleep, mood and, energy levels.

Once the initial detox feelings pass from eating too many nutrient-dead carbs (or, just too many carbs period) you may find that your brain fog lifts as well as your energy. Your digestive issues may ease and your sleep may improve. You might notice that your eyes look brighter and your skin is clearer. I see and hear about these changes in my clients all the time.

Then, something else might happen...

You might go to the other extreme. You might experiment with eating too few carbs. This could happen because once you start to NOURISH yourself daily, you won't be starving all the time. Eating enough calories daily, filled with protein, healthy fats, and low-sugar, fibre-rich carbohydrates may actually *decrease* your appetite—you may not be hungry. And, one of the things that happen when people cut way back on their carbs is that they lose some weight on the scale. For people looking to lose weight, this feels like a major coup!

Trust me, it's not.

But, because you like the way you are feeling, you might think less is more and cut back on your carbs even further. Beware of this! Anytime I review a client's food log and see that they are averaging less than 50 grams of carbs per day, I urge them to reevaluate their goals. Recall what I said at the start of NOURISH about the fact that any diet will create change. The questions are is the diet healthy and can you sustain eating the diet for life?

In my experience, most people can only withstand a very low carbohydrate diet for a limited amount of time. And then, when they go back to eating even a more moderate level of carbohydrates, the body fights back by storing excess fat and water, the guts protest with digestive issues, sleep is not restorative, the mind returns to monkey mind chaos and energy levels go up and down.

Many of your old issues might reappear…

Again, the Scale Can Lie. STAY OFF THE SCALE.

Weight loss on the scale from not eating enough carbs is likely just from water loss. And, weight loss on the scale when people eat too few calories or fast for extended periods of time could be from lean muscle mass loss. This is not good! As we age, we want to work to keep lean muscle mass not sabotage ourselves to lose more of it by making rookie mistakes like eating too few carbs or not enough calories or protein.

Your Optimal Grams of Carbs Per Day

Do the initial work using TAAP so you can discover your optimal grams of carbohydrates a day. Otherwise you could be destined to stay on the magical misery tour of dieting. You could remain high in body fat with low in energy and chronic digestive issues. You could continue to be plagued by sleeplessness and fluctuating moods. You might stay underweight and unintentionally starving!

You want to choose high-fibre, low-sugar, carbohydrates and the **Game Changers** chapters will teach you how to do just that. Let's talk about the first game changer: fibre.

CHAPTER FIFTEEN

The doctor of the future will no longer treat the human frame with drugs,
but rather will cure and prevent disease with nutrition.
— Thomas Edison

Game Changer Number One: Fibre

One of the reasons I asked you to track your water intake when you started NOURISH was to prepare you to *slowly* increase your fibre intake. Water will help to prevent digestive issues that may arise like constipation, bloating, gas, or diarrhea when you begin to gradually increase your fibre grams per day. TAAP to find your tipping point for fibre and you may find that your digestion levels off.

For my clients, I use the Mayo Clinic guidelines as a baseline for minimums. I challenge women to see if they can get their fibre up to **20 grams per day** and men up to **30 grams per day**[23]. One reason to increase fibre is to help improve digestive regularity. You want to get your guts moving! Again, you will learn from TAAP what your best number of fibre grams is per day. Pay attention to your digestion, your sleep, your mood and your energy levels as you ADJUST your fibre intake.

Fibre Requirements	Age 50 or younger	Age 51 or older
Men	38 grams	30 grams
Women	25 grams	21 grams

I ignored getting enough fibre at the beginning. My high-sugar carbs were my only source of fibre. I had to try alternatives, like flax and hemp seed. I now include fibre with almost every meal.

— Jessica, NOURISH client

Upon reviewing client's food logs, I see a trend of extremely low fibre consumption—often under 10 grams per day—for both sexes. And, when I ask about digestion, most people have issues of some sort. They are either chronically constipated or they have diarrhea or they flip-flop between the two. Also, foul-smelling gas and bloating is an embarrassing problem for many people.

If you have been eating a very low fibre diet—20 grams per day or less—make sure to gradually increase your fibre grams per day. Do not go from consuming six grams of fibre per day to 36 grams per day the first week or you could experience digestive distress. Add more fibre to your diet slowly. For example, you could start by adding three to five extra grams over the course of several days. Then, use TAAP to see how you feel. ADJUST your fibre up or down, bit by bit, gram by gram, to find your tipping point. How much fibre per day keeps your digestion running smoothly for you? How is your energy? How is your skin? And, always pay attention to your sleep and your mood too.

I was shocked about how little fibre I was getting into my system! Loving vegetables and always being mindful of including high-fibre foods (supposedly) in my diet, it stunned me to see how little it was really amounting to [when] I TRACKed my food.

—Rebecca, NOURISH client

Why Do We Need Fibre?

Our guts are filled with bacteria—both good and bad. The good bacteria loves fibre; the bad bacteria loves sugar. Colonies of good bacteria help to keep our immune systems healthy and our hormones in check. Too much bad bacteria makes us sick, too thin, or over fat and cranky.[24] If we are eating a fibre-less, high sugar diet, we're not taking care of our guts. It's that simple.

Think about your digestion. Are you irregular? Do you have bowel movements several times a day, like a puppy? (Eat. Poop. Eat. Poop.) Or, do you have movements more like three times per week? What is normal for you? Constipated one day and loose the next? Do you have gas that scares your partner? Do you fear going out for dinner because of not being able to get to the toilet in time? Maybe you think, *my guts are just slow,* or *I have a nervous stomach.* But have you ever thought about why your guts are slow? Or, about why you have a nervous stomach? It could be you need more water daily. It could be due to the fibre-less, nutrient-dead food that you have been consuming. There is a saying that fast food is fibre-less food. Guess what? Some seemingly healthy, fibre-rich foods are full of dead carbs and sugar. Cereal and granola bar eaters, beware!

Remember: bad gut bacteria—the kind that makes us sick—loves sugar!

Eating too little fibre (and too much sugar!) can make us store body fat, give us an overactive monkey mind, and can make us depressed, hyperactive, or listless and craving-ridden. When you decrease your sugar intake and increase your water and your fibre, digestion often levels off. With a digestive tract that is functioning well, you can potentially see improvements to your health like your digestive distresses ease or are eliminated completely. Your energy levels could rise and your body composition (fat to muscle ratio) might improve. Your immune system might get a boost along with your mood. You might notice that the quality of your sleep is enhanced and that your blood chemistry improves (cholesterol and blood sugar levels regulate). Your skin might get clearer.

It is possible to consume too much fibre.

Consuming too much fibre will carry nutrients out of the body before they can be used to your advantage. Too much fibre without enough water can also make you constipated. As well, too much fibre can make you too loose. This is one of the reasons you need to make sure you are drinking enough water daily.[25] It is also another reason why you need to TAAP. If you have a smart phone, make sure that fibre is one of the categories showing on the app screen so you can keep TRACK throughout the day. When you find fibre sources that work well for you, proactively log them ahead of time. Experiment with how much fibre works for you. You can only learn this if you TRACK, ASSESS and, ADJUST.

I have female clients who do really well on .21 grams of fibre per day; I personally need 25 to 28 grams per day. I have men who feel great on 35 grams per day and others who notice a positive change if they stay around 40 grams of fibre per day. In my thirties, I needed between 35 and 38 grams of fibre per day! Things change and so must your nutrition and you won't know unless you TAAP. Here is the challenge: you need low-sugar fibre sources.

Fibre Sources:
- hemp seeds*
- flax seeds (ground)*
- avocados*
- cacao nibs*
- chia seeds (whole or ground)*
- psyllium husks
- nuts and seeds (walnuts, macadamia nuts, almonds, sesame and pumpkin seeds)*
- coconut (unsweetened)*
- sprouts – *alfalfa*
- olives*

*As well as offering low-sugar, fibre sources, these foods will increase your healthy fat levels and up your calories proactively to meet your BMR and your TDEE daily caloric ranges.

It is time to reconsider some traditional fibre sources that might not be serving you. Basically, this means all of those foods that are nutrient-dead or *full of sugar!* Some examples are fibre bars, bran cereals, granola bars (glorified candy bars) and unlimited, high-sugar fruits.

Always ask, what am I hungry for? And, what am I getting for what I am eating?

Go back and review your food logs:

> What was your highest day for grams of fibre?
> What was your lowest day for grams of fibre?
> What was your fibre grams average for the week?

Gradually add in more fibre and keep drinking your water. Get curious, read labels, and try new things. Again, do this slowly. Don't run to the store and buy everything on the list! Not only is this a needless expense, adding too many new foods to your diet at once can be stressful for the body. If you have never been inside a health food store, now is the time to go. Bring the list of recommended fibre-rich, low-sugar foods with you to the bulk food store and stock up on a few items at a time. You have the rest of your life to experiment—there is no need to do this all at once. Also, you might try hemp seeds and love them while you may not care for cacao nibs. That's ok! You won't know what works for you until you give some of these foods a whirl. It is time to find your nutritional tipping point for your daily fibre intake. When you do, you will begin to see changes in things like your appetite,your digestion, your sleep, your mood, your body composition, your skin and, your sex drive.

The second game changer, sugar, is up next.

CHAPTER SIXTEEN

We are addicted to a low-fat, high sugar diet as alcoholics are to alcohol, because high Insulin levels create the same brain state that alcohol does.
—TS Wiley

Game Changer Number TWO: S–U–G–A–R
Sugar is a Nutrient-Dead Substance

The American Heart Association links eating too much sugar to multiple health issues, including heart disease, obesity, and high blood pressure.[26] For many of us, the sugar game plays out in our bodies like this…We eat sugar. It tastes good.

We feel good because of the dopamine release (the feel good hormone). We want more sugar. We lose the sugar high. We get the "hangries"—we're hungry and angry. We store unwanted body fat. We want more sugar.[27]

Imagine the drug addict trying to kick his habit and at every corner there is a convenience store that offers as many drugs as he can consume! The stores serve up drugs that are cheap and readily available in all flavours, textures, and colours. If you are a sugar addict heading out into the world, you haven't got a chance. We are talking about table sugar (sucrose), high-fructose corn syrup (which is in everything from pop to pop tarts to yogurt), and fructose (fruit sugar). Fructose has been touted as safe and is in all of our kids' snack foods. However, just because fructose doesn't raise blood sugar levels and Insulin immediately does not mean that it is not doing possible damage in the long run.[28]

When my daughter was little and I didn't understand how serious the effects of sugar—even natural sugar like fructose in fruit—could be, she had juice every day. I also fed her things like fibre-rich granola bars instead of cookies and cakes, thinking that these were healthier choices. Even though she ate enough protein every day, she was always starving! She would eat cereal and orange juice for breakfast and sandwiches for lunch. For dinner, if she ate macaroni and cheese she would tell me she was still hungry twenty minutes later!

It turned out that she was hungry. My daughter was starving in fact, for more healthy fats, *less* sugar and *more* fibre.

The best nutrition choice I ever made for my family was to stop buying juice. Doing so helped to wean us off the magical misery tour of the sugar game. You too could be perpetually nutritionally bankrupt if you live on fast, cheap food or if you are mistakenly under nourishing yourself with nutrient-dead "health food." Make the decision to stop buying processed foods today. If you don't and you choose to keep nutrient-dead junk in your house, you or someone you love will eat it. Guaranteed.

Sugar and carbs really did a job on me! I did not know until I started ASSESSing my sugar. I find that I am calmer now and don't have as many hot flashes. I also experience less anxiety now that my sugar and carbs are under control.

–Layla, NOURISH client

Group	Sugar intake (grams)	Sugar intake (teaspoons)
Women	24 grams	6
Men	36 grams	9
Teenagers	20–32 grams	5–8
Children 4–8	12 grams	3
Preschoolers	16 grams	4

The chart above refers to the American Heart Association's recommendations for daily intake of added sugars[29]. For NOURISH, I want you to TRACK and ASSESS *all sugar*—including the sugar in fruits and vegetables. Even if you are not adding in table sugar, there is sugar in many of the foods we eat. You can easily TRACK your sugar on the nutrient tracking app. (Make sure you have included sugar in your display settings if you have a smart phone.) This week, start reading labels and wean yourself down to 36 grams of sugar per day for men or 24 grams of sugar per day for women[30]—or less. Begin to make nutritional choices that meet your daily optimal range for carbohydrates while watching your sugar intake. Then, use the TAAP system to check in with your compass questions. As you wean yourself down to consuming less sugar per day, ASSESS your sleep, your digestion, your mood and, your energy level? Always ask, *What am I hungry for?* And, *What am I getting for what I am eating?*

Remember, eat what you want when you want, but TAAP. ASSESS what are you getting for what you choose to eat.

Instead of flavoured yogurt, I add my own berries—this allows me to be in control of the amount of sugar I eat. Simple little changes like that made a big difference for me.

–Avery, NOURISH client

We have discussed how too many carbs and excess sugar (and too little fibre) disrupts us hormonally and affects our body composition and our brains. But what else does it do? For me, too many carbs (above my 100 grams per day maximum), too little fibre (below 25 grams or above 38 grams) or too much sugar (for me, above 16 grams per day) makes me sleepless. I wake up tired and feeling hung over. I end up bloated and retain non-essential body water. This means my face is puffy, there are ring marks on my hands, and sock lines on my ankles.

And I am incredibly body sore.

What I get when I eat too many carbs and too much sugar is pain, both muscularly and in my joints. I also get the pain of the annoyance from mental assaults from my monkey mind when I go beyond my nutritional tipping points. For me, it's just not worth it.

What about you? What do you get back from eating a carb-heavy diet that is fibre-less and laden with too much sugar?

Sugar had been feeding the unwanted guests in my body (bad bacteria, yeast and mould) for years. I was in a serious case of denial, I guess.
—Trina, NOURISH client

What About Fruit?

Hands down, the biggest issue clients have with cutting back on sugar is fruit.

"But, what about my fruit?" they ask.

My question back is: "But what if all that fruit is keeping you fat, 'hangry,' sleepless, and wasted?"

I am not suggesting you never eat fruit. I eat fruit every day. I am suggesting that you continually ask yourself: *What am I hungry for?* And, *What am I getting for what I am eating?* Ask whether the things you are putting in your mouth are building you up or tearing you down. Because make no mistake— everything you put in your mouth is doing one or the other.

Consider how that morning banana benefits you. ASSESS how you feel after you have an apple as your mid-morning snack. How much sugar is in those mangoes you toss into your protein shake? See if that orange in the afternoon satisfies you until dinner. Looking more closely at your daily sugar intake requires that you stop being a passenger on the magical misery tour in terms of your nutrition. Instead, stick with TAAP and TRACK, ASSESS, ADJUST, and PROGRESS.

I hated having my coffee without sugar for the first two weeks. Now if someone gives me one with any amount of sugar in it, I cannot drink it.
—Ed, NOURISH client

Names for Sugar

Always read labels on everything you eat. Here are some other names for S-U-G-A-R:

- agave
- barley malt
- beet sugar
- brown rice syrup
- brown sugar
- buttered sugar
- cane juice
- cane juice crystals
- cane sugar
- caramel
- carob syrup
- caster sugar
- coconut sugar
- confectioner's sugar
- corn sweetener
- corn syrup
- corn syrup solids
- crystalline fructose
- date sugar
- demerara sugar
- dextran
- dextrose
- diastatic malt
- diatase
- ethyl maltol
- evaporated cane juice
- fructose (fruit sugar)
- fruit juice concentrates
- galactose
- glucose
- golden sugar
- golden syrup
- high-fructose corn syrup

- honey
- invert sugar
- lactose
- malt syrup
- maltodextrin
- maltose
- maple syrup
- molasses syrup
- muscovado sugar
- organic raw sugar
- oat syrup
- panela
- panocha
- polydextrose
- rice bran syrup
- rice syrup
- sorghum
- sorghum syrup
- sorbitol
- sucralose (Splenda)
- sucrose (white table sugar)
- sugar
- syrup
- treacle
- tapioca syrup
- turbinado sugar
- yellow sugar[31]

As a recovering alcoholic, NOURISH helped me quit my latest addiction—sugar. Initially that was my biggest surprise, just how toxic sugar is. And sugar is hidden everywhere.

–Dinah, NOURISH client

Work (and yes, it is work) to wean your sugar grams to 36 grams a day for men and 24 grams a day a day for women. You're still TAAPing to find your nutritional tipping points. Remember that too much sugar may be making you fat, hungry, anxious, sleepless, PMS, sexless and wasted. And, sugar leaves you empty…Get really clear on what nutrient you need now and IF the sugar content of that food is worth it based on the other nutrients offered. For example, is that stale, brownie Sunday at the chain food restaurant really worth the digestion distress and sleeplessness it will cause you? Is that cereal that is full of sugar worth all of the carbohydrates with little to no grams of fibre?

Remember in the protein chapter I said not to get stuck in a rut of eating protein all day long? The same is true if you are a fruit-a-holic or a baby carrot connoisseur. Learn to watch your sugar intake in everything you consume.

Look at the nutritional values of each of the fruits below:

Sample Food Log (fruit)							
	Prot (g)	Fat (g)	Sat (g)	Carbs (g)	Sugar (g)	Fibre (g)	Cals (kcal)
Item							
Apples 1 medium	0.36	0.23	0.039	19.06	14.34	3.3	72
Avocado 1 medium	4.02	29.47	4.273	17.15	1.33	13.5	322
Banana 1 medium	1.29	0.39	0.132	26.95	14.43	3.1	105
Clementine 2 medium	1.42	0.25	0	20	13	4	79
Kiwi 1 medium	0.87	0.4	0.022	11.14	6.83	2.3	46
Raspberries 3/4 cup	1.11	0.6	0.018	11.01	4.08	6	48
Pear 1 medium	0.63	0.2	0.01	25.66	16.27	5.1	96
Grapes (red or green) 1 cup	1.15	0.26	0.086	28.96	24.77	1.4	110

Compare the sugar content of the apple versus the avocado. Now, look at the fibre content of each. Next, look at the healthy fat content of each. Traditional thinking, teaching, and dieting have people freaked out about the calories and fat in avocados! So, people choose the apple—and load up on sugar. Recall what was advised previously: not more than 36 grams of sugar for men and not more than 24 grams per day of sugar for women. There are 14.34 grams of sugar in an apple!

To me, this is a no-brainer—I want the nutrient-rich avocado for the healthy fat and fibre and the low sugar. After I eat an apple, an hour later I'm starving. If I have an avocado, I'm good to go for hours. And, avocados are a fruit!

Note: Again, if you are not accustomed to eating high fibre foods, go slowly! For example, there is over 10 grams of fibre in an avocado! If you have been consuming a diet very low in fibre and you suddenly eat a whole avocado, you could end up with bloating, gas, constipated or with diarrhea.

Next, look at the sugar in vegetables. Which should you eat more of, and which might you want to cut back on?

Sample Food Log (vegetable)							
	Prot (g)	Fat (g)	Sat (g)	Carbs (g)	Sugar (g)	Fibre (g)	Cals (kcal)
Item							
Broccoli 1 cup chopped	2.57	0.34	0.035	6.04	1.55	2.4	31
Carrots 1 cup chopped	1.19	0.31	0.047	12.26	5.81	3.6	52
Cauliflower 1 cup chopped	1.98	0.1	0.032	5.3	2.4	2.5	25
Spring Mix (lettuce) 2 cups	1	0	0	4	0.9	2	20
Beets 1 cup chopped	2.19	0.23	0.037	13	9.19	3.8	58
Celery 1 cup chopped	1.24	0.24	0.06	6.02	3.56	2.4	27
Asparagus 1 medium	2.95	0.16	0.062	5.2	2.52	2.8	27
Green Beans 1 cup	2	0.13	0.029	7.84	1.54	3.7	34

When you make these changes, you may be satisfied with just regular, nutrient-rich meals. You may not feel that you need to snack every couple of hours. And, remember, you won't know unless you TRACK, ASSESS, and ADJUST. That is how you PROGRESS.

Review Your Food Logs

What was your highest day for grams of sugar?
What was your lowest day for grams of sugar?
What was your sugar grams average for the week?

Surprised? Remember, men are shooting for 36 grams of sugar per day (or less) and women are aiming for 24 grams of sugar per day (or less). Do you start your day full of sugar? If the answer is yes, are you starving by mid morning?

A reminder, on NOURISH, if you are hungry, eat! But always ask, *What am I hungry for?* And, *What am I getting for what I am eating?* Make sure to TRACK everything you put into your mouth.

Cutting down on sugar was an enormous benefit for me. Knowing that I have to keep my daily sugar intake under 24g is huge because of my candida (yeast) issue. I have more energy, I feel better, and I'm more at peace with myself when I lay off sugar.

—Trina, NOURISH client

Continue to TRACK and now focus on ASSESSing and AD-JUSTing to find your nutritional tipping points. Maybe your digestion is better drinking three and a half litres of water a day. Maybe you train hard in your workouts and need to up your protein. Perhaps you are consuming too much protein and should swap your Greek yogurt for regular yogurt to cut back on your protein consumption. Maybe you find you cannot resist eating a whole container of macadamia nuts and should stop buying them. It's time to do things like check the label on those "healthy crackers" and see what you are getting nutritionally from them. Could you be satisfied with a half a cup of berries instead of a full cup to cut back on sugar? Could you try an avocado if you never have? Yes. You can do all of these things and more to create self-care habits that serve you.

Look at your food logs nutrient numbers and aim for the guidelines as outlined in NOURISH. Focus on the macornu-trients: protein, fats and carbohydrates. Don't forget the two game changers fibre and sugar. Remember, if we don't TAAP, we're guessing. Perhaps guessing is what brought you to NOURISH in the first place? Keep TRACKing your food and ASSESSing the nutrients. Make ADJUSTments to find your nutritional tipping points to PROGRESS.

CHAPTER SEVENTEEN

Sugar is the devil, and fat isn't making me fat! Who knew?
—Tanya Drain

CHECK IN, ASSESS and ADJUST

You now have all of the nutrition information for NOUR-ISH. Are you using it? How are you feeling? Have you been asking the questions what am I hungry for and what am I getting for what I am eating?

Welcome to the ASSESS Part of NOURISH

This chapter is about checking in and remaining curious by asking and answering ASSESSment questions. Asking and answering questions is very important on the journey towards finding your nutritional tipping points. It's time to hone in on what foods make you feel sluggish and grouchy, or make your face break out and give you digestive distress. Limit these foods in your diet or eliminate them entirely. It's also time to notice what foods make you feel energized, calm, and clear headed. Eat more of them! We cannot know unless we TRACK, ASSESS, and then ADJUST our food choices to make PROGRESS.

Check In: Ask the Four ASSESSment Questions

Rate your answers to the three questions on a scale of 1 to 10 (1 = poor; 10 = excellent):

How is my digestion? Why?
How is my sleep? Why?
How is my mood? Why?
How is my energy? Why?

Are your numbers to the questions maintaining? Improving?

Preplan your days so you know which nutrients are lacking and fix it! Your body works with what you put in it. If you eat garbage, you will feel like garbage.

–Layla, NOURISH client

What could you be doing better? (List)
What are you doing well? (List)
Are you meeting your daily caloric needs?
Are you eating at your minimum grams of protein per day?
Are you consuming healthy fats every day?
Which new healthy fat sources have you added to your diet?
Are you considering your carbohydrate sources and making smart carb choices?
Are you consuming 36 grams (or less) of sugar per day if you are a man and 24 grams of sugar per day (or less) if you are a woman?

I am recognizing how my food relates to my mood. If I get over my sugar limit, my mind starts to race—the monkey mind takes over. For example, I had to go to a birthday party yesterday and saw the difference in how I felt after eating cake and ice cream. I never would have realized this before starting NOURISH.

–Abigail, NOURISH client

Are you eating enough fibre?
Have you hit your fibre grams per day tipping point yet? And, if so, how do you know?
Have you been to the health food store yet to pick up some healthy fat and fibre sources to add to your daily nutrient-rich intake?
What new fibre sources have you added to your diet?

While my body was seeing a transformation, my thought process was also changing. I acknowledged how food affected my moods, whether it was celebratory or stress relief. I also made excuses for my bad eating habits, finding ways to justify them. I stopped blaming others for my bad food and beverage choices. I started seeing benefits other than just looking good.

–Jessica, NOURISH client

Here are a few more questions to ask:

Is something you are eating regularly making you bloat?

Do you sneeze, cough or clear your throat every time you consume specific foods or drinks?

Are you congested after you eat certain foods?

Do you get ring and sock lines when you don't drink enough water?

Does too much sugar give you a headache? Make you hyper? Lethargic? Sleepless? Does too much sugar increase the number and intensity of night sweats?

Start to Focus on the *ADJUST* Part of TAAP

Assignment

Review your answers to the questions above and begin to make ADJUSTments in order to PROGRESS. Always ask: *What am I hungry for?* And, *What am I getting for what I am eating?*

CHAPTER EIGHTEEN

A well-spent day brings happy sleep.
–Leonardo da Vinci

SLEEP: Lights Out for Sleep

I was an insomniac for almost 20 years. I tried everything to get some zzz's. You name the sleeping medication, and I tried it. Although nothing seemed to work, desperate, I remained curious and kept searching. Finally, the answer to my sleeplessness came in this cocktail: I changed my food, I stopped over-exercising and I shut out the lights.

Studies show that the body sleeps better in total darkness. We are just designed that way. Any light in our bedrooms can disrupt our sleep.[32] That means light from things like alarm clocks, cell phones, night lights, hall lights, street lamps, flood lights and, light that creeps under closed doors.

Making the choice to sleep in the dark is not news for many insomniacs. My husband and I have slept in total darkness for years. But I came across some serious reminders while doing nutrition research relating to sleep habits. Sleeping in total darkness was stressed over and over again to get adequate sleep. Is your bedroom truly as dark as you can get it?

Beware of light coming from under the door(s). We leave the light on in the kitchen downstairs. I realized that light seeps up the stairs and under our bedroom door. We swapped that light for the laundry room light instead, and that made a huge difference.

Turn your phone or alarm clock over and put it on the floor. This was huge for us. No more blue/green glow all night long! Phones and clocks live on the floor, lights down. What a huge difference!

Add another window treatment. We have blinds in our bedroom windows that are 100 per cent light blocking. However, we also have a yard light that works from dusk until dawn. Although the blinds were custom fit for our window, it is not totally flush to the sides of the window frame. The glow from the yard light slips in through the sides of the blind, and that light keeps our room illuminated. I bought light-blocking drapes for the window, and now the room is in complete darkness. After our first night in total darkness, we both woke up amazed at the profound difference.

Wean your kids off the night-lights. If your kids won't go cold turkey, do this over time. Kids love to learn about their bodies. Take the time to educate them about how important sleep is for their health. Make sleeping in the dark fun and about staying healthy instead of something to be feared. Stress that sleeping in darkness helps to regenerate their growing bodies. Suggest that they will be faster and smarter if they sleep in the dark.

Never ever give up on your quest for sleep. Sleeplessness can be attributed to many health ailments, including depression, weight gain, irritability, low energy, anxiety, weight loss, and hormonal issues.[33] Stay curious and keep searching for the answer to a good night's sleep.

Additional Considerations to Improve Sleep

Consider what you are eating for your last feeding of the day. TRACK, ASSESS, and ADJUST if sugary desserts, alcohol or caffeine keep you tossing and turning. If you wake up starving in the middle of the night, consider a fat, fibre, and protein snack before bedtime. A tablespoon of almond butter is an excellent choice.

Also, if you drink alcohol at night and experience disruption in your sleep, ask yourself if it is worth it. Do certain alcoholic drinks affect you more than others? For example, for me, wine is a killer. Wine leaves me sleepless and fat-storing if I drink it on a regular basis. And, think about your water consumption...Are you spreading your drinking water out through the day or are you consuming the vast majority of it in the afternoon and evening? I have many clients in the health-care and beauty industries. I also have a lot of clients who are teachers. Many of them complain that there is no time to drink water during the day. Almost all of them choose to compensate by hydrating after hours instead. And almost all of them are up during the night to pee. Listen to yourself: *No time to drink water?* That is silly.

Don't forget about sleep hygiene! Change your sheets. There is nothing like fresh, crisp, clean linens. Buy the best sheets you can afford and change them often. Sanitary sleeping conditions can make a huge difference in your sleep. It's a good idea to keep the bedroom cool too. Sleeping in a cool room helps to lower the body's core temperature and allows for better sleep. You can try adding some white noise. We sleep with a fan on year round. Or, try earplugs and buy a sleep mask. Shop around; there is a mask out there that will be comfortable for you. Don't be fooled by price. I've had great masks from specialty stores that I paid a premium for and right now my mask came from the drugstore.

Stay curious, keep searching, and do not underestimate the power of your nutrition and how it relates to your sleep.

Questions

Have you ever suffered from insomnia?
If yes, why?
Do you sleep in the dark?
If you have kids, do they sleep well?

CHAPTER NINETEEN

Being entirely honest with oneself is a good exercise.
–Sigmund Freud

What About Exercise?

You have begun the NOURISH program in earnest. You need to work out too, right? Physical fitness is an essential element of your health and wellness. Exercise is good for the heart (cardio), builds lean muscle mass (strength training), helps to maintain joint health (stretching), and aids in keeping or improving on our balance as we age. The old adage "use it or lose it" is true. We need to keep moving. Exercise also plays a major role in proactive stress management and brain health. Plus, exercise makes us feel good!

As a coach, I see many people abuse exercise. This abuse stems from a misunderstanding of how exercise works in the body. Most people turn to exercise because they think it will make them thinner or they believe it will rid them of their stress. If you believe you can outrun the cheeseburger, fries, and shake that you grabbed on the way home because you are too stressed out and busy to cook at home, and if you think you can do hundreds of crunches to flatten your abs—you are mistaken. With the popularity of extreme (and main-stream) high-intensity interval training, the inclination to punish our bodies into submission can be all consuming:

You're over fat, you're out of shape, and you're sick of it. Why not begin with that late-night, infomercial, extreme exercise DVD set you bought for New Year's that you haven't even unwrapped? Or, just start running. How hard can that be? Runners are thin, right? Maybe start with hot yoga and sweat it all out. That will work, right?

Before You Punish Pause

For many of us, the temptation to start pounding the heck out of ourselves as soon as we've had enough is compelling. It makes sense, right? We're trained to believe that those of us who have made our own slothful beds deserve to be hammered back into shape. But before you thrash, I would encourage you to pause, take a breath, and consider this: taking a body that is out of shape, under NOURISHed (even if it is overfed), possibly starving, sleep deprived, and stressed to the max and beating it into a pulp with hard-core exercise is not going to help.

In fact, it could make things worse.

Besides injury, more stress, and eventual failure, erupting into an extreme exercise routine could even make you more fat or cause you to *lose* lean muscle mass. Yes, that's right. Exercise without properly NOURISHing yourself could make you lighter on the scale only because you are losing muscle!

Before starting an exercise program, I recommend to all of my non-exercising nutrition clients that they give their bodies six weeks to ADJUST to the changes they have made in their food. Remember, stress is stress. First, we all have to earn the right to progress...

I signed-up for NOURISH because I am 38 and had been working out hard for eight months. I could not figure out why I could not lose the love handles or the extra weight in my chest area; I could not get rid of my man boobs. And, the less I ate and the more I exercised, the fatter I got. This was so frustrating! I knew deep down it was my food. After only a few weeks on NOURISH, the man boobs started to shrink, my energy was back, and I started sleeping through the night.

–Ed, NOURISH client

Start Here

NOURISH. Make sure you are well fed with nutrient rich foods that serve you before starting an exercise regime. If when you started NOURISH, you were not exercising regularly, wait six weeks before adding exercise into your self-care routine. Walking, stretching, restorative yoga, Tai Chi and Chi Gong are fine. But, nothing with more intensity than that for the first six weeks. If you are already an avid exerciser, I still recommend keeping your routine the same while you AD-JUST to the protocol of NOURISH.

Next, focus on sleep. If you are not sleeping, focus on gentle exercises like walking and stretching. Do not take a tired body and stress it more by adding in high intensity exercise like running or boot camps.

Breathe. That's right. Check in to see if you are actually breathing deeply enough to oxygenate your brain and NOURISH your body. Practice three minutes of conscious breathing daily to help to manage stress, encourage sleep, and energize you. And, I encourage you to forget about belly breathing. Our lungs are in our chests! So, breathe deeply into the top of your lungs—right up to your collarbones, in between your shoulder blades and into the nape of your neck. Exhale completely and make sure to rid your lungs of old, stale air before re-oxygenating yourself with a full, deep breath.

Move. Your body is an amazing machine; move it thoughtfully. The cool, hard-core, bragging-rights exercise can come later. Just walk, stretch, play outside with your kids, go for a stroll with your neighbour's dog—anything. If you sit at work, consider getting a standing desk. Or, if you must sit, set your alarm to remind you to get up and move very hour. Whatever you do, make sure to move your body daily. The body is designed to be in motion unless it is sleeping.

A Note About R-U-N-N-I-N-G

Running is something that many people think they should start doing once they embark on making healthier lifestyle choices. If you love to run and it comes naturally to you, your body composition is where you want it to be, and you sleep well and are injury-free—keep running. If you have tried running and stuck with it for a period of time (say six months or longer), you have proper shoes, you have had your form checked by someone who knows more than you do (e.g. a professional—not your neighbour) and you suffer from things like foot pain, back pain, knee pain, neck pain, weight gain, sleeplessness, anxiety and, countless other ailments …

It is okay to stick a fork in your running career. Some alternatives for distance running are high intensity interval training (HIIT), walking or running up hills, sprints, and, walking.

A lot of people turn to running because it's free, seems relatively easy, and they think it will make them thinner. It might, but probably not. Anyone and everyone can try running, but not everyone should continue to run.

Reasons to Use Your Running Shoes for Something Else

You have joint issues. Although weight-bearing exercises are important for maintaining lean muscle mass and building bone density, people with joint issues may not need the pounding of running.

You are obese. People who are obese might consider strength training and walking over running (for potentially far better fat-loss results too!).

You hate it. People who can't stand running should *stop running!* Exercise should be something you can tolerate even if you don't love it.

There's one more thing, and this one is the most important: Maybe it's time to ask: *What am I running from?*

High Intensity Style Exercise

If you want to incorporate high intensity interval training workouts, make sure to focus on thoughtful, intentional exercise. Have a coach who understands **proper form and technique**. Anyone can hang their shingle out after a weekend course and call himself or herself a trainer. Find someone with experience to guide you safely.

Remember, we have to earn the right to progress. If your body chronically hurts from any exercise you are doing or you find yourself getting injured frequently, stop. Speak with your doctor and your trainer about possible solutions. Finally, although working out is important, you will improve your health faster and further by learning how to properly feed yourself than with exercise.

READER'S NOTES:

PART III:
Cooking

CHAPTER TWENTY

If you can read, you can cook!
–Murdo MacDonald, M.D.

If You Can Read, You Can Cook!

First, notice that this is a chapter about cooking and not a recipe chapter. In my experience with my nutrition coaching clients, I've found that if they can cook, they get curious about how to ADJUST recipes to meet their nutritional requirements based on the lessons in NOURISH that have helped them to find their nutritional tipping points. And, if *you* can cook, you will do the same. If you know how to cook, you may find the section below on substitutions helpful.

Sometimes clients say, "I'm bored with healthy food." But, the truth is, they were eating the same food *all the time* before they started to eat healthfully. Think about it. You probably were too. It is true that they are not making any new meats, healthy fats and oils or vegetables and fruits any time soon. And, the food industry is busy coaxing us into buying things like pretzel-crusted, cheese, and tortilla-chip-loaded, frozen "dinners." Resist! Stick to real, nutrient rich foods that serve you instead and make it yourself.

Healthy People Cook

Again, the truth is, healthy people eat the same foods all the time. If you get bored with healthy food choices, try some new recipes. If you can't cook, a chapter full of recipes won't make any difference. If you are new to cooking read on...

My grandfather used to say, *If you can read, you can cook!* I sometimes come across people who are embarrassed because they don't know how to cook. Often these people are parents or heads of households. They know that they should not be feeding their family out of a box but they never learned to cook as kids and as time went by they were too ashamed to ask for help, let alone take a cooking course.

I get it.

I was 28 before I learned how to cook. I lucked out when an equestrian client of mine wanted to barter for her horseback riding lessons. She was a professional chef and in exchange for riding lessons, she gave me a weekly cooking lesson. I also paid her a weekly stipend for groceries and ate dinner with her and her family her five nights a week. Now, over 15 years later, I love to cook. And, I am still learning...

Years ago, I used to offer a *Kitchen Basics* course for nutrition clients who did not know how to cook. We went over how to use knives and how to roast chicken breasts and vegetables. Now, I offer them two things: Google and YouTube

Seriously. Today, everything you need is right at your fingertips! And, healthy food does not need to be complicated food. Let me say it again:

Healthy people eat the same foods, all the time.

And, if you can read, you can cook.

There is no getting around it—if you want to be healthy, you *must* cook. What's great about this? If you're reading this, you can read a recipe. And, in today's technological world, recipes are just a click away. Also, recall the chapter **Get Over Your Self. Get Started!** where I talked about how most of our excuses are just fear? And, remember what I said about most of us learning what we know about food from our parents or caretakers? The same thing is true about cooking. Just because your mom was a lousy cook doesn't mean you have to be one too.

You have probably realized by now that I am not going to give you a meal plan. There are no fridge lists in NOURISH. Other than vegetable oils and trans fats, I don't even tell you what *not to eat.* I only ask that everything you put in your mouth, you TAAP. I do offer you a few charts with low carbohydrates fruits and vegetables to consider and there is a list of possible "new to you" fibre choices to find at the bulk food or health food store. But, that's it.

I'm not going to give you a recipe chapter.

If you want new chicken recipes, try Googling "grain-free chicken recipes." If all you can come up with is gluten-free pasta, chicken Alfredo, get curious. Could you use zucchini noodles for the pasta to add more nutrition with less carbs? The same thing goes for desserts. Do you really need Agave syrup and brown sugar and honey in your dessert? If you are someone who has a chronic sweet tooth, it may be subject to change once you wean yourself off copious amounts of sugar—both added and natural. Ask yourself about your sweet tooth. Are you craving sweets because you're still eating low fat? Why are you still eating low fat if it is not working for you? Try mixing up a half-cup of organic raspberries, two tablespoons of heavy cream and a tablespoon of ground chia seeds and eat up! Voilà! A dessert with protein, fats, healthy carbs and fibre that is low in sugar.

What I am going to do is give you some substitutions and tips that helped my clients and me make both choosing and cooking NOURISHing foods more user friendly.

Substitutions

Make sure to save these in the nutrition tracking app as a favourite meal for easy reference.

Cereal: Mix up some of your healthy fibre choices like flax, chia, shredded, unsweetened coconut and pumpkin seeds, add in some heavy cream and a touch of salt and cinnamon to taste. If you prefer hemp seeds to pumpkin, use them instead. If you like both—throw them both in! If you want warm cereal, heat it up. Voila! Healthy cereal.

Bread: Use cabbage and Romaine lettuce leaves instead of pita bread. Google almond flour bread and flax wraps and raw wraps. Try making homemade wraps savory by adding herbs such as paprika, onion powder, and garlic powder, or sweet with cinnamon or nutmeg.

Salad: Are you sick of salad? Chop up low-sugar, phytonutri-ent-rich veggies. Make a huge batch, and you'll have enough for the whole week. Be creative. Kids love this too! Add feta and it's suddenly Greek. Add Jack cheese and stir in some salsa, and a dollop of sour cream and it's Mexican. Throw chia and flax in to up the fibre and healthy fats. Try sprinkling in some goat cheese and walnuts and add some balsamic vinegar.

Dressings and Sauces:

> Use sour cream instead of mayonnaise.
>
> Use coconut sauce (also called coconut aminos) instead of soy sauce.
>
> Use almond butter instead of peanut butter for "peanut" sauce.
>
> Use almond or coconut milk.
>
> For lighter oil in dressings, try walnut or avacado.
>
> Lemon juice and salt and pepper—simple and delicious ingredients for a quick dressing on any salad.

Substitution for Starches: Google how to make cauliflower rice or cauliflower mashed potatoes. Both are excellent substitutions for rice and potatoes. You can add them to any-thing—eat them plain or season as you would the "real thing."

That's really it. That's what we who are NOURISHed do. You can absolutely make this process of figuring out your nutritional tipping points and how to cook very complicated. Or, you can stay curious and get creative. *Always ask what am I hungry for?* And, *What am I getting for what I am eating.* And, Google. Happy cooking!

READER'S NOTES:

PART III:
The Halfway Point
ASSESSment

CHAPTER TWENTY-ONE

All happiness depends on courage and work.
–Honoré de Balzac

You've Got This, Right?

Remember, you have all of the nutrition information for NOURISH right now. Are you getting this? TAAP: TRACK, ASSESS, and ADJUST, to PROGRESS. That's all you have to do. Accountability is part of the practice portion of NOURISH. You are practicing; you are still a work in progress. When the 12 weeks are over, yours skills to maintain your accountability habit—to yourself—will be honed.

If you never had to ASSESS, there would be no point in the program. The ASSESSing is how you learn to establish your own nutritional tipping points. For example, maybe you need 21 grams of fibre instead of 32. Perhaps you should eat regular, full fat yogurt instead of Greek to cut back on protein. Maybe you function best on three and a half litres of water on your workout days. These are examples of how you might ASSESS and ADJUST your tipping points. After years of research and experimentation and years of eating this way, I have my own tipping points figured out.

And, I still ASSESS and ADJUST regularly.

That is because life changes all the time. Circle back to the list in the chapter **Get Over Yourself. Get Started!** You will take that cruise, your kids will go off to school, the holidays will come every year and your spouse may or may not be on board with NOURISH. You picked up this book to help your self. TAAP is how you do it! Put some thought and energy into your ASSESSments. Make the ADJUSTments required. Do this for yourself.

ASSESS your food logs weekly, every Sunday on or before 9 PM—not Monday morning or Tuesday afternoon. How we do one thing is how we do everything. This principle applies to feeding ourselves. Blowing off the weekly food log ASSESSment exercise is actually blowing off yourself and quite possibly, your well-being. You can do this. Remember that you are *learning*. Do the work and the results will follow.

NOURISH client Carol explains: "As a person who is 'off the wagon' more than on, sticking with TAAP feels much better than being off. Last week was an extremely busy week for me personally and professionally, and I was exhausted. On the weekend, I reflected on why I was feeling so drained. My schedule was busy, yes, but it came down to poor organization, which led to dehydration and poor nutrition choices that in the end just caught up to me. I can't eat rice crackers, a piece of cheese, and one protein shake (and nothing else) and think that I can maintain my energy."

Poor nutrition and poor planning for me means low energy, anxiety, craving empty carbs, irritability, poor digestion and feeling physically drained.

After three days back into TAAP:

I feel lighter.

I am less bloated.

I sleep soundly.

I feel rested in the morning.

I am less irritable.

I have less brain fog.

My mood is better and I'm just happier.

How About You? Are You TAAPing? Are You Asking: What am I Hungry For? And, What Am I Getting for What I Am Eating?

My personal mantra is: keep the water and fibre up, and keep the sugar down.

–Bonnie, NOURISH client

Ask the Four ASSESSment Questions:
1. How is your digestion?

What is your number from 1 to 10 now? Are you having bowel movements every day, at least once? Seriously. Check your bowel movements and ASSESS Are your bowel movements non-foul smelling? Are they light in colour? Do your bowel movements float? Are they non-greasy? Are your bowel movements free of undigested food particles? Are you gassy? Are you bloated? Are you constipated? Are your bowels loose? Are you a little of both—constipated and loose? .

Then ask, how is your water intake? Are you drinking 64 or more ounces of water a day? If not, why not? How is your fibre consumption? Are you consuming enough low-sugar, fibre per day? If not, why not?

I never really felt like I had an issue with digestion. But when I went into self-sabotage mode one day partway through the program (after I had been doing well), I was blown away at how the poor food choices I made affected me. It was a day of substituting what was right [with] what was convenient. I felt terrible for two days after. Lesson learned.

–Trina, NOURISH client

2. How is your sleep?

What is your number from 1 to 10 now? Are you falling asleep easily? Are you staying asleep? Are you waking up rested? Are you sleeping in complete darkness? If not, why not?

Ask and answer these questions too: Are you eating enough calories? If not, why not? Are you considering how caffeine and alcohol affects you? If not, why not? Have you cut back on sugar? If not, why? Are you eating 34 grams of sugar or less per day (men) or 24 grams of sugar or less per day (women)? If not, why not? If yes, what changes do you notice? List them:

Because I am paying attention through TAAP—TRACKing and ASSESSing—I now know I need to limit my caffeine to two cups of coffee per day and have them before nine in the morning.

–Abigail, NOURISH client

When I started really looking at my sugar intake and got my numbers down below 36 grams per day, I finally slept through the night for the first time in years. Now, if I want to sleep, I know now that I cannot have a high-sugar dessert at night (like raspberry pie) or I will not sleep. It's a choice for me now—sleep or pie. Nine times out of ten I choose sleep, because rest gives me more than a piece of pie ever will.

–Ed, NOURISH client

3. How is your mood?

What is your number from 1 to 10 now?
Is your monkey mind in check?
Is your outlook positive?
Are you less moody?
Are you less depressed?
Are you less anxious?
Are you happier?
Are you experiencing no change? If yes, why?

TRACKing my nutrients, ASSESSing them and then—ADJUSTing them has helped me to finally get off my anxiety medication. I had no idea how my food was affecting me until I kept track and paid attention to how I am feeling. Keeping a daily log of my moods really helped me to see the light.

–Daphne, NOURISH client

4. How is your energy?

What is your number from 1 to 10 now?
More energy?
Calmer?
No change? If yes, why?

Are You TAAPing?

TRACK: Are you tracking *everything* that you put into your mouth? Honestly? Explain:

ASSESS: Are you evaluating your food logs? Really? Or, are you still waiting to be told what to eat and when? Explain:

I love learning that it is possible to get your numbers right without completely sacrificing the food that you enjoy!

–Kelly, NOURISH client

You need to ASSESS in order to learn how to feed yourself (and your family/partner/people you love) in a way that serves you. You are a work in progress. Decide ASSESS proactively. Preplan your nutrition. Become *proactive* instead of *reactive*.

Example: Proactive (Adult)

"Tomorrow is a busy day of meetings for me. I better pack some nuts in my bag and organize my water bottles tonight. As well, I plan on having a great, protein, healthy fats and fibre-rich, and low-sugar breakfast, so I can skip the lousy food offerings at the meeting. Plus, I'm going to hard-boil some eggs, too, so when I get home I can have an egg while I cook dinner."

Example: Reactive (Child/Victim)

"I did it again! I really didn't eat well today. But they didn't give us very healthy choices, so all I could do was eat the veggies and the unhealthy dips. Then, I was starving after work and had to stop at the coffee shop for a bagel and cream cheese and a coffee with two sugars, and then I knew I had used up all of my calories for the day, so I skipped dinner. Now, I'm plugging my food into the nutrition tracking app because Cait wants me to, and I'm awake in the middle of the night because of the late afternoon caffeine, and because I didn't eat nutrient-rich food because I didn't plan, because I need other people to take care of me and offer me the proper food choices, because I am too childlike about taking care of myself. So, I am over fat/skinny-fat/wired/tired (fill in the appropriate term) and not very pleased with myself. Again."

Which one are you? Proactive or reactive? Explain:

Here is another "aha" halfway moment from NOURISH client Carol: "I learned that you can't discuss nutrition with just anyone. Although I love my friends, they serve me in different ways; with some friends I would never choose to discuss nutrition, as we are not always on the same page when it comes to this subject and this can lead to sabotaging."

ADJUST: Are you making changes?

Are you staying curious? Are you shopping several times per week for produce? Are you seeking out new fibre sources? Are you doing things like hard-boiling eggs every week?
Are you using a water-logging app? Are you cooking protein in bulk at least two days per week? Have you been to the bulk or health food store? Are your veggies washed, cut up and ready to go? Have you switched to full-fat dairy? Have you tried different kinds of nuts? Are you using things like sour cream instead of mayo? Have you tried new oils like walnut or avocado to use in salad dressings? Are you making your own sauces and salad dressings?

Have you changed the settings on the nutrient tracking app to focus on what you need for this program? For example, if eating enough fibre is still an issue but you have your protein figured out, can you swap one for the other on the settings? Or, can you swap fats for sugar? Have you emptied your house of all of the non-nutritive junk that is poisoning (yes, that's correct) you and your family?

I track the crap too—this is key! Seeing the numbers beside the foods that are not ideal for me helps me to be accountable.
                                                    –Bethany, NOURISH client

"But, It's So Hard!"

Really ask yourself this question. How hard is this? Remember what I said in the **If You Can Read, You Can Cook!** chapter? You can make this hard and slip into a state of overwhelm but, will that help you? If it feels like a lot, remember—*you're learning*. Remind yourself that "hard" is spending time and energy at the doctor's office and spending money at the drug store. Suffering from digestive issues is hard. Having kids who are sick (all of the time) because you don't feed them well—that's hard. (You do buy the groceries, right?)And, so is:

- getting diabetes
- having a heart attack
- having a stroke
- not being able to play with your kids, grandkids, nieces and nephews, your dog, etc.
- having no sex drive
- having nothing to wear because nothing fits OR nothing feels good on you
- enduring chronic headaches
- suffering from PMS
- succumbing to moodiness
- having a four-season, chronic cold
- having bad skin
- eyes that are dull and lifeless
- hair that is dry and brittle

Having a low self-esteem and faking it is hard. And, so is not doing things in life because you're too thin, too fat, over-tired, wired, depressed, unhappy, worn out and,used up.

Those things are hard. Living well is all about making healthy choices.

PROGRESS: TRACK, ASSESS, ADJUST, to PROGRESS

It is time to go back and reread the nutrition lessons. Really soak on what I have asked you to think about in terms of the nutrient-rich foods you are putting into your body. Percolate on the lessons. Be honest. What are your nutritional tipping points? What are your averages for protein, fats, carbohydrates, sugar and fibre? What are your getting for what you are eating?

Here is NOURISH client Dinah's note from the halfway point in the program:

"Early on, I think I was overwhelmed—it is a lot of information to take in. I needed to be easier on myself. This is a process, and it was helpful to look at it as such. I didn't realize how much I was victimizing myself. I'm not a victim, nor do I want to portray that kind of energy. What I'm getting is education to improve my (and my family's) health, and in turn, my life. The biggest thing I've learned so far is how ignorant I was about nutrition! I'm learning that fibre is my new best friend, and that I have been setting my daughter up for failure with the foods I'm packing in her lunch. I'm making PROGRESS with my sugar consumption (and my mood when I eat too much sugar—sugar is like vodka for me). I'm making progress trying different things so I can meet my daily goals (especially in fibre and protein).A behaviour that doesn't serve me is the "poor me's." I can get into that mood pretty quickly and can start beating myself up. I am working on stopping this behaviour. To stop this, I will do two things I remember you said:

"When I told you that I don't eat well when my husband doesn't cook for me, you said, 'What are you, five?'

"Instead of thinking of the things I'm giving up or missing out on, I'm going to think about all the things I'm gaining."

Ask...

What is working well? (List)
What could you be doing better? (List)
What are you learning? (List)
Are you making progress? If so, what exactly? (List)
Are you stuck in a victim's mindset? If so, why? (List)
Are you the king or queen of self-sabotage? How?

Jessica's halfway progress report...

"I'm working on exceeding my BMR by eating a minimum of 1800 calories per day. I finally gave up diet pop (it took a couple of weeks, but today is day four!). I'm keeping my carbs in the 75 to 100 range and introducing more healthy fats. I'm averaging 60 to 80 grams of protein per day. I will do more pre-planning my meals and snacks and posting the day's meal plan in the nutrient tracking app in the morning to see where I need to increase or decrease nutrients proactively. I will schedule lunches instead of saying I am too busy to eat. I'll do more mid-week shopping and bulk cooking, and using spices instead of sugar-based sauces. I will TRACK my water and not just guessing that I have had eight glasses."

What About You?

What can you do to stop behaviours that don't serve you? List them. And, reflect back on what you want to get out of this program? What are you still hoping for? Has it happened yet? How will you know when you get there? Will you continue to do the work required? Why or why not?

Justine's food log halfway through the program:

Sample Food Log Week #5	Prot (g)	Fat (g)	Sat (g)	Carbs (g)	Sugar (g)	Fibre (g)	Cals (kcal)
Breakfast							
Butter 1/4 tbsp	0.03	2.88	1.824	0	0	0	25
Egg 2 large	12.58	9.94	3.099	0.77	0.77	0	147
Bacon 5 slices uncooked	12	18	7	0		0	220
Coconut Oil 1 tbsp	0	13.6	11.764	0	0	0	117
Total	24.61	44.42	23.687	0.77	0.77	0	509
Lunch							
Cherry Tomatoes 10 cherry	1	0.27	0.063	7	4	2	30
Cheddar Cheese 2 cubic inch	8.47	11.27	7.171	0.44	0.18	0	137
Cucumber 1/2 cup chopped	0.39	0.11	0.009	1.44	0.92	0.5	8
Chicken Pepperoni 1 sausage	7	2.5	1	1			50
Total	16.86	14.15	8.243	9.88	5.1	2.5	225
Dinner							
Olive Oil 2 tbsp	0	27	3.728	0	0	0	239
Green String Beans 1 cup	2	0.13	0.029	7.84	1.54	3.7	34
Chicken Breast 100 grams	22	1	0.1	1	1	0	105
Sweet Potato 60 grams	0.94	0.03	0.011	12.07	2.51	1.8	52
Total	24.94	28.16	3.868	20.91	5.5	5.05	430
Snacks/Other							
Raspberries 1 cup	1.48	0.8	0.023	14.69	5.44	8	64
Macadamia Nuts 2 ounces (10-12 nuts)	4.48	42.96	6.839	7.84	2.59	4.9	407
Total	5.96	43.76	6.862	22.53	8.03	12.9	471
Total	72.36	130.49	42.66	54.09	19.4	20.45	1635

Justine made progress! She ate a more moderate amount of protein, more healthy fats, she made time for lunch and her calories are at least meeting her BMR minimum.

What About You? Are You Making Progress?

Finally, what chapter of the poem *Autobiography in Five Chapters* are you on now?

Autobiography in Five Short Chapters
−By Portia Nelson

1.
I walk down the street.
There is a deep hole in the sidewalk.
I fall in.
I am lost ... I am hopeless.
It isn't my fault.
It takes forever to find a way out.

2.
I walk down the same street.
There is a deep hole in the sidewalk.
I pretend I don't see it.
I fall in again.
I can't believe I am in the same place.
But it isn't my fault.
It still takes a long time to get out.

3.
I walk down the same street.
There is a deep hole in the sidewalk.
I see it is there.
I still fall in ... it's a habit.
My eyes are open.
I know where I am.
It is my fault.
I get out immediately.

4.
I walk down the same street.
There is a deep hole in the sidewalk.
I walk around it.

5.
I walk down another street.

Start of NOURISH: Chapter_____   **Halfway:** Chapter_____

Halfway Metrics

If you are at the six-week mark of NOURISH, it is time to take your second set of metrics. Go back to the instructions and the charts in the **Your Starting Point** chapter and take your second round of measurements, metrics, and photographs.

A major motivator for me was seeing the difference in the pictures between my first and second metrics. After that, I kept asking my friends if they wanted to see pictures of my sugar-free ass!
                                                        –Dinah, NOURISH client

The good news is you have all of the information you need to take massive action towards a healthier you. **The next six weeks is when the magic happens.** This is when your body will start to believe that you will NOURISH it on a consistent basis. You just need to go do it.

READER'S NOTES:

PART V:
The Stories

CHAPTER TWENTY-TWO

The Case Studies: The Core of NOURISH

Until I started writing this book, I taught the information for NOURISH in person, face to face, with clients. I saw these men, women, and children on a weekly basis—sometimes three to four days per week. I saw them for an hour and a half on the night of their nutrition coaching course, every week for six weeks, and at their fitness classes or in their private personal training sessions with me.

Our mutual desire to learn and create positive change—along with our collective curiosity and humour—is what made NOURISH so effective for so many. To recreate this alchemy, I asked clients to contribute their stories to NOURISH. In this part of NOURISH, you will find their journeys laid out in their own words. These are not Olympic athletes, movie stars, or people with personal chefs. The case studies are filled with people who are students, who work for a living, who are raising families, or who are navigating through retirement.

They range in age from 11 to 68 years old. Some of these people are very fit and some do not exercise (and may never). The cream of NOURISH is the stories of the people who helped to create it. I am grateful to these people for sharing their experiences.

Note: Use the table below to understand the Case Studies' body fat percentages. Body fat percentages are calculated based on age, body weight, and body fat calliper measurements. These calculations help you to understand how much of your body weight on the scale is lean mass (muscle, water, bones, blood, and organs) and how much is actual fat. As you scan people's body fat results, make sure to look at their lean muscle gain relative to their fat loss. Notice how, in many cases, actual weight loss on the scale was marginal. In some cases, clients *gained* weight on the scale. This is because they gained lean muscle mass. Muscle weighs more than fat—but it takes up less room. This means that people went down pants, dress, and shirt sizes. Or, if they were too lean, by the end of NOURISH their clothes fit better—they did not hang off their bodies.

Body Fat Categories		
Category	Women (% fat)	Men (% fat)
Essential Fat	10–13	2–5
Athletic	14–20	6–13
Fit	21–24	14–17
Acceptable	23–31	18–25
Obese	32+	26+

READER'S NOTES:

Case Study Stories: Six Weeks

CASE STUDY 1 (six weeks)
The Correctional Officer: Justine's Story

Age: 38
Height: 5'7"
Activity Level: currently a non-exerciser
Goal: To regulate my hormones, improve my mood, increase my energy, lose body fat, and increase muscle tone.

METRIC	START	6 WEEKS	TOTAL
Body Fat %	20.77	15.24	−5.53
Lean Pounds	120.43	122.90	+2.47
Fat Pounds	31.57	22.10	−9.47
Weight	152	145	−7

I decided to see what the NOURISH program was all about when I reached a point in my life where I felt like I was losing control. I wasn't overweight, or even unhealthy in the eyes of most, but I was not happy. I was at a point in my life where I was very low energy, my mood was all over the place, and I was sick and tired of always feeling sick and tired. While working a full-time job, married to a shift worker, and a mother of three active children, I had difficulty finding the time to figure it all out.

When I started working with Cait, the first task was to TRACK everything I was eating. At first, this was a challenge for me, as I was eager to start making change, and I was somewhat embarrassed of all the "quick meals" we were consuming. As I went through the early stages of NOURISH, I realized how important it was to see exactly where my problem areas were. Making small changes the first couple of weeks resulted in huge changes in how I was feeling, and [I] continued to improve. I didn't realize how much fruit I was eating and how much sugar I was consuming—I thought that having a banana was better than having a chocolate bar.

I can't believe how my eating habits have changed in the last six weeks, and how much better I feel when I follow the principles of NOURISH and TAAP I am now at the point where I ASSESS my own food logs to see what I need to keep doing and where I need to improve. It is all about changing your mindset about what you eat. I used to be a constant snacker, but now I am amazed at how little I feel the need to constantly eat. I have recognized the importance of planning, and my house runs more smoothly when we know what we are eating.

There are so many resources out there about nutrition! It gets confusing. NOURISH lays out in a no-nonsense way what needs to be done to feel better. The beauty is that rather than giving meal plans and specific things to eat (which seems handy at first) you go through NOURISH as a learning process and through TAAP (and trial and error), you see what works to meet your goals and what does not. I realize it is not about perfection, rather about making progress, which is a much more realistic goal for me.

CASE STUDY 2 (six weeks)

The Grandmother: Bonnie's Story

Age: 55

Height: 5'3"

Activity Level: one Pilates class, one yoga class, one high-intensity interval training per week

Goal: Continue to enjoy my life into my old age by staying active and eating well.

METRIC	START	6 WEEKS	TOTAL
Body Fat %	31.40	24.34	−7.06
Lean Pounds	98.79	105.92	+7.13
Fat Pounds	45.21	34.08	−11.13
Weight	144	140	−4

I have always been interested in maintaining health through exercise and nutrition for both my family and myself. Staying at home to raise two children involved in competitive sports, food was always prepared at home for trips to the local rink, tournaments, and so on, in an effort to provide the nutrients needed for our active lifestyle. I always knew the importance of food choices and exercise and enjoyed working out at the local gym. I had always been lean, many would say skinny, and I am often described as a wee peanut.

My nutrition journey started in earnest around age 50. Around that time I started to see noticeable changes in my body; I just seemed to be getting thicker. Many life changes occurred at the same time; my kids left home, I returned to school and then started working full-time, and I became a grandmother—exciting stuff indeed! Through it all, I continued to focus on what I thought were healthy food and lifestyle choices, but with less positive results.

I participated in the NOURISH course not once, but twice. Why twice? Simply because there was so much to learn! This is an entirely different way of eating and literally flies in the face of what is most commonly believed to be right. Make sure to read and re-read the lessons often.

CASE STUDY 3 (six weeks)
The Life-Long Dieter: Lucinda's Story

Age: 60
Height: 5'2"
Activity Level: Pilates class and yoga class, once a week
Goal: To improve my self-esteem and quality of life.

METRIC	START	6 WEEKS	TOTAL
Body Fat %	25.96	21.55	−4.41
Lean Pounds	116.98	121.60	+4.62
Fat Pounds	41.02	33.40	−7.62
Weight	158	155	−3

When I was 10, my Dad told me he would give me a dollar for every pound I lost. That was when I started down the yo-yo diet trail. Every diet I was on was "the best." But, I would lose weight, go off the diet plan and gain the weight back. I never learnt how to properly eat. I just learnt what not to eat to lose weight. One plan I was on was 600 to 800 calories. I lost and lost big. But, once again, when I quit the diet, I gained all the weight back and more.

What did eating healthy look like? I did NOT know.

In September 2014, I was feeling overweight, out of shape and I was about to turn 60. I thought I better get my life in order. My fresh start began with an email to Cait.

I had tried so many diets and eating plans but I trusted Cait; I knew that NOURISH was what I wanted to try. The next session was starting in March, my birthday month. I thought this would be my birthday present to myself.

I got my metrics done, my pictures and was instructed to TRACK everything I ate. "Don't change a thing," Cait said. "Just TRACK everything you eat to establish your baseline." Well hallelujah! When I started, it was the week of my 60th birthday. There was lots of eating out and friends inviting me for a drink. As instructed, I did TRACK, I did eat, and I did drink...

After receiving back my food log with her comments on it...I still was not getting what I wanted. What should I EAT? Low carb, low fat, low whatever! I just wanted Cait to tell me what you do.

She didn't.

So, I TRACKed. I read the lessons on the macronutrients. I read and reread the lessons on fibre and sugar.

"Now, ASSESS," Cait said.

I had never taken the time to ASSESS how I was feeling let alone what I was eating and what it was doing to me. I had been having heart palpitations for a while. I didn't stop and think about it or worry. But, I did now...And, I worried about what I should eat, and that I did not sleep, and, and, and...I started acknowledging how I felt by thinking about my digestion, my sleep, my mood and my energy. Then, I made ADJUSTments.

I adjusted my food entries to get my calories up. I had never eaten this many calories unless I was "off my diet" and binging! Now I was curious. Who eats all these fats and loses weight? But, Cait reminded me, "You need to eat fat to lose fat."

Previously, I didn't eat fiber because it made me constipated. But, when I included more fibre, I started to feel better. And, the less sugar I ate, the less monkey mind I experienced. And, my heart palpitation were starting to subside...I reviewed my food log and noticed that Cait asked about the amount of Green Tea I was drinking daily. I started to finish all of my caffeine before noon. And then, I started sleeping better. Other things like my indigestion improved and food cravings stopped. I was not losing weight on the scale, but my clothes fit better.

On the day of my six-week metrics, I awoke excited and nervous. I had completely changed the way I ate. I changed the way I thought about certain foods. I had logged my food faithfully for six weeks. I felt amazing—younger with more energy. It was no wonder! I was finally sleeping and I was less moody. People started noticing a change in me. My skin was softer, my eyes were sparkling, and my hair was shinier. I felt great! People asked, "What have you done Lucinda? You look amazing." I would answer, "Looking after myself and eating healthfully." Because, finally, I really was.

It is totally true that you are what you eat.

Back to my six-week metrics…My six-week metric appointment opened my eyes to understand success in a different way and not by the scale. At the appointment, the scale didn't move much, but the other measurements told the story. I was amazed at the numbers!

Then we looked at my photograph at the start and then six week into the program. Wow. The photos were the proof I needed that this program—this way of eating—was working. It was good for me. And, I learnt it was okay to eat an occasional cookie, a drink a glass of wine. I just had to TRACK, ASSESS and ADJUST accordingly to keep making PROGRESS.

I now have the strength to stop at one cookie, or four, chocolate covered blueberries, and, not feel guilty. Slowly, I am erasing any old thoughts. Thoughts like that I am bad for eating a "forbidden food." On NOURISH, nothing is forbidden. I can eat whatever food I want. I just need to TRACK, ASSESS, and get back on my routine.

Every day on NOURISH just gets easier and easier. I still am learning. I like to TRACK as it is a time for me to reflect, not only on what I eat, but how I am feeling and what I want to achieve. Instead of reacting, I am being proactive. This gives me so much power to make good choices and ADJUST not only what I eat, but also what I do and how I feel about it.

NOURISH has been so much more than just a journey about food for me. This has been a 'stop and smell the roses' moment for me.

CASE STUDY 4 (six weeks)
The Retired Civil Servant: Abigail's Story

Age: 68
Height: 5'5"
Activity Level: weight training twice per week, moderate
Goal: Enjoy my retirement, improve my self-esteem, outlook, and well-being.

METRIC	START	6 WEEKS	TOTAL
Body Fat %	36.79	33.11	−3.68
Lean Pounds	151.60	155.18	+3.58
Fat Pounds	88.30	76.82	−11.48
Weight	240	232	−8

I have to admit that I began my nutritional journey looking for a confirmation of what I had been doing, not very successfully. I assumed a refresh would assist me to go at it again. I had tried almost every diet imaginable. Boy, was I in for quite a different kind of journey, complete with a whole new way of looking at food and me. While I was anxious to concentrate on exercise, Cait slowed me down and asked me to consider that nutrition was at the core of a great variety of the challenges that had been facing me. Not only that, but she introduced me to what, at the outset, seemed like a complex set of understandings on nutrition-rich foods. She asked me to be patient, experiment with foods, and build my knowledge so that I was acting in an informed way about my food choices.

So, I started down a new [path].

The more she talked to me, the more I went back and researched old understandings and the science behind what she was now telling me. Many of the beliefs I had were based on old and poor research and had been replaced with new views. As I looked at each macronutrient—protein, fat and carbohydrate, and especially the two game changers, fibre and sugar—I learned new facts, replaced erroneous ones, and headed forward. I started to see the old patterns and [swapped] them with new ones that resulted in a stronger, healthier, and happier me. Gone were my feelings of guilt; relinquished were the "should haves," and in their place was an optimistic sense of progress and making decisions in a mindful way. I began sleeping better, my knees stopped aching, my muscle tone improved, and I felt I was walking taller and stronger.

The key to making NOURISH work in my mind is to TRACK every day in terms of food and exercise. I had many excuses over a lifetime of why I didn't need to TRACK. But, I now see that it is the only way to stay on course. I find it very helpful, not only to ASSESS what I have been doing but, more importantly, to ADJUST my plan for future days. Nothing is left to one's imagination—it is laid out. If one TAAPs the results follow. And with all the different tools it is that much easier to complete.

I know I am only at the beginning. The real work will continue each and every day, but I know I will be a success because I am patient in my learning, mindful in my food choices, and accepting of the need to continue evaluating results as I move forward.

CASE STUDY 5 (six weeks)
The Soldier: Adam's Story
Age: 39
Height: 5'11"
Activity Level: currently not exercising, focusing on nutrition for first six weeks
Goal: To manage my PTSD and become more proactive about my health.

METRIC	START	6 WEEKS	TOTAL
Body Fat %	21.14	17.59	−3.55
Lean Pounds	195.57	204.38	+8.81
Fat Pounds	52.43	43.62	−8.81
Weight	248	248	0

As I sit here attempting to find the words to describe why I chose to take the NOURISH program, I am reminded of my former self. I am a retired member of the Canadian Armed Forces who served 10 years in the Armoured Corps as a reconnaissance soldier, who has been diagnosed with Post Traumatic Stress Disorder (PTSD) and struggles with the transition from military life to that of the civilian world. I was also diagnosed with a disease called Sarcoidosis two and half years ago, for which I take a steroid called prednisone to help my body regulate the inflammation that affects my lungs and all of my major organs. Above all else I am a husband, a father, a son and a brother, who is constantly seeking to discover my true and authentic self.

I have struggled with finding my place in this world upon leaving the military and have wandered in and out of many career paths during the last nine years and I feel that I have finally found my calling. I have recently graduated from a Social Service Worker program at a local community college and will begin my Bachelor of Social Work degree this coming fall. It turns out that I really enjoy working with people and learning about how I can better this world one conversation at a time. This realization left me looking in the mirror at a reflection of somebody that I used to know, because like most people who attempt to help others, we often neglect ourselves in the process. I chose to take the NOURISH program because I need to start thinking about my well-being and myself for a change.

I must be honest that I was hesitant in the beginning of this program and constantly told myself that I was doing this for my wife and children because they needed me to change and be better. I accepted no responsibility for my decision to start this program and because of this train of thought I did not feel completely committed. I realize now that I was lying to myself right from the start and only time and the courage to be honest with myself would allow me the opportunity to begin my transformation into the new me, the real me.

On NOURISH, I made positive food choices and learned about how much control and strength I can achieve by simply TRACKing my food. I maintain positive levels (for me) of protein, fats, carbs fibre and sugar. I have learned that I love fibre. Before I started the NOURISH program I thought that I was eating well and that my food habits were not too bad. But, one week into NOURISH and I realized that I was starving myself! I was surprised by how little food I was consuming and by how many of my calories came from negative or empty caloric sources. Within one week of the program I realized the importance of healthy eating habits and that connection to my overall well being. I think it is safe to say that I was fully committed at this point, because once you know how good you can feel, you can never "un-know," and really, why would you want to forget?

I have discovered that I am in control of the food I eat and it does not hold any power or control over me. I have also learned what the word "moderation" actually means and the importance of it. But most of all I have learned not to be too hard on myself and to realize that I am worth every moment of happiness that I am given in this world. I would like to share a few words that I wrote at the half-way check in point of NOURISH:

"I am making lots of progress, both in physical appearance and in mindset. I have discovered that by making positive choices in my food habits I have the ability to fuel myself for success. I have discovered that change occurs organically if you give it a chance and stay open to the possibilities that can occur when you view your life through a different, more informed lens, with your health and happiness as the only desired outcome. I have made progress in allowing me to think of me."

Wow.

Now I am filled with a sense of hope for what the future holds for me and accomplishment for the positive choices I have made over my journey through the NOURISH program. If someone had told me years ago that I could gain control over my life by making positive choices with my food I would have laughed at them and called them a liar. I now realize how wrong I would have been. I would like to state that I am sleeping better than I ever have and feel that I am happier and more focused because of the NOURISH program. I think that this program has the ability to become the foundation for personal growth and discovery, and it can empower people to take control over their lives and become their true and authentic selves.

Case Study Stories: 12 Weeks or longer

CASE STUDY 6 (12 weeks)
The Entrepreneur: Kelly's Story

Age: 38
Height: 5'4"
Activity Level: high intensity interval training twice per week
Goal: To manage my monkey mind, improve my sleep and digestion and level off my moods.

METRIC	START	12 WEEKS	TOTAL
Body Fat %	7.84	7.27	−0.57
Lean Pounds	106.91	114.98	+8.07
Fat Pounds	9.09	9.02	−0.07
Weight	116	124	+8

As someone who has always been on the lean side, I never thought much about what I ate. My mantra was: "I eat what I want, but I watch what I eat."

I always ate healthfully—lots of fruits and vegetables, very little pre-packaged food, no pop, no fast food, and only the occasional treats. But, I never TRACKed what I ate to see the breakdown of what I was putting in my body. I had no idea if I was really getting what I needed.

On NOURISH, I learned from TAAP that I was eating 200+ carbs a day, and around 50-75g of sugar (mostly from fruit). My fiber was all over the place and I had no idea how much fat I should be eating. I didn't think about it because I had so little fat on my body.

But, this is how I was feeling: I was tired all the time; no matter how much sleep I got I never felt rested. I just attributed this to my three kids. I was cranky. I had no patience—again, my kids' fault. I was emotional, which I thought was my husband's fault, because he worked on the road. And, my digestion was awful! I was either bloated or had stomachaches and was constantly irregular. Plus, I could not shut off my monkey mind at night. I would wake up and then be awake for hours.

I never thought that it was my diet that was making me feel this way because there was always another excuse—my kids woke me up seven times last night, my husband is away, my kid is sick, I am bored of being a stay at home mom etc.

Then life changed.

I bought a business, my kids started sleeping through the night (for the most part), my husband was home. I wondered, gee, why wasn't I feeling better? Oh wait; maybe it's my diet! So I started TRACKing what I ate and the improvements I have seen are undeniable. If I wake up during the night, I can go back to sleep (no monkey mind), if I still feel hungry at the end of the day I know it's because my carbs are too low (which for me is under 100 because I am naturally very lean—a true ectomorph body type—I can tolerate more carbs). I also know that my fiber intake has to be between 25 and 30 or there are adverse affects. If I eat too much sugar I feel hung over in the morning and I am short tempered. Bloating is a a direct result of too much sugar and the wrong type of carbs. Healthy fats (like avocado and nuts) satisfy me. I can tell when I haven't eaten them for a day or two.

My body now craves foods that are NOURISHing my body and actually "feeding" me not just "filling" me up. I don't "need" to eat 2200 calories a day anymore. If I am eating the right kind of food I can feel satisfied at 1800-1900 calories a day.

Has my body changed that much? Not really. I am up a little in fat (not a bad thing) and I am up a bit in muscle (also not a bad thing). Do I look healthier? I think so! And my photographs prove it. My state of mind and overall wellness (as well as my family's) have definitely reaped the benefits of NOURISH.

CASE STUDY 7 (12 weeks)
The Retired IT: Kevin's Story

Age: 60
Height: 5'10"
Activity Level: avid exerciser, active golfer
Goal: To age well and maintain an active lifestyle.
And, to improve my golf and curling games!

METRIC	START	12 WEEKS	TOTAL
Body Fat %	5.71	8.27	+2.56
Lean Pounds	140.50	138.52	−1.98
Fat Pounds	8.50	12.48	+3.98
Weight	149	151	+2

First, let me offer some background about me. I am retired with lots of time on my hands and I enjoy trying out new ideas or trends. So, with no real "axe to grind," I decided to experiment with my eating habits to see what, if any, improvements I could make.

I was already exercising one to two times per week. I was curious to see what might happen to my body in terms of improved muscle tone and strength if my diet focused on a few specific areas. The Internet was full of "answers" and "studies" many of which seemed to contradict the other. I tried juicing (green and otherwise), smoothies, and attempts at reducing my carb intake that resulted in a feeble attempt at the Ketogenic diet (consuming below 50 grams of carbs per day). The results were mixed. I TRACKed my food intake using an on-line app, but I was not sure how many carbs or how much protein to consume or which fats were good or bad. During this time, my digestive system was somewhat unstable as I experimented with different amounts and types of foods.

I decided I needed to gain a better understanding of what my body really needed. I was losing weight, but I didn't want to lose muscle mass as well. Cait had an opening in her nutrition coaching course, NOURISH, so the timing was perfect. This was to be a three-month experiment, or so I thought...

NOURISH emphasized the importance of TRACKing and ASSESSsing what I ate. Since I had been TRACKing my food for the past few months, I knew what I was putting into my body at the start of the program. I thought I was eating healthfully. What a surprise to learn that my regular breakfast of banana, bran cereal, and low fat cream had more sugar than I needed for the whole day! And, the bigger surprise was that healthier choices could include eggs, full fat dairy (who doesn't love heavy cream?), and bacon. I was hooked!

Throughout NOURISH, ADJUSTing to full fat, lower carb meals with a daily caloric intake over 2800, involved pre-planning meals and increased trips to the grocery stores for fresh produce. During that time, my body was constantly re-acting (some days better than others) to the different foods I was ingesting. After one particularly unintended "full cleanse," I was a little skeptical if I was doing the right thing by subjecting my digestive system to this regime. But things improved quickly as I continued to make better food choices. Thanks to a supportive wife, we emptied the cupboards of the bad processed foods and leftover Christmas treats. I strongly recommend that anyone doing the NOURISH program remove all temptations!

With the information provided in NOURISH and the TAAP system, my eating habits are now focused on nutritional tipping point specifically for me. Along the way, I learned to look at and question the nutritional labels on processed foods. What an eye opener! I have reduced or eliminated all grain based breads, pasta, fruit juices, pies, and most other foods with high sugar or starch content. Surprisingly, I don't miss those foods. I have replaced them with copious amounts of leafy vegetables, berries, full fat everything including cheese, nuts, and seeds (I discovered how good hemp and pumpkin seeds are) and lots of water. I eat all types of meat and fish. I am eating more than before I started the program!

The rewards for this journey are too many to list, but here are a few:

Physically I have more energy and stamina than ever. Keeping up with others half my age at exercise classes is definitely an ego boost! I have less body fat (waist size decreased two inches, love handles gone) and new clothes that fit well. I have noticeable increased muscle tone and digestion patterns that I understand and can control. Plus, I sleep better.

Emotionally I am calmer and experience less moodiness—no more highs and lows.

Mentally my thinking is clear. And, I feel younger and not tired (turning 60 is not a limiting number). I receive many positive comments from friends and family who try to emulate my eating habits and are always questioning what I eat and looking to try it themselves.

What was intended to be a three-month personal experiment with nutrition instead turned into a lifelong and, hopefully, long life journey of healthy food choices. There's no need to turn back.

CASE STUDY 8 (12 weeks)
The Triathlete: Ruby's Story
Age: 50
Height: 5'4"
Activity Level: high-intensity interval training two
times per week, yoga class one time per week, horse-
back riding
Goal: To age gracefully and get rid of my muffin top!

METRIC	START	12 WEEKS	TOTAL
Body Fat %	24.89	17.64	−7.25
Lean Pounds	130.70	133.42	+2.72
Fat Pounds	43.30	28.58	−14.72
Weight	174	162	−12

I am 50. I am telling you this because it is important to know
that I have been around the block over the years [trying] all
the diet and nutrition fads as my got-to-be-skinny tools. Before NOURISH, I felt like I was floating around, needing a
change but not knowing what the change needed to be.

Through NOURISH, I realized that no one can do it for
you—there is no magic Band-Aid. I do not want to eat in a
way that makes me feel hungry or suffer from cravings.
And, being skinny is not the goal, and being skinny won't
make things right.

When I decided to try NOURISH, I was looking for a
way to change the way I looked at food and eating. What I
learned is that you cannot get rid of your cravings until you

give the body what it needs. I had to give my body what it was actually craving: more healthy fats, more fibre and more calories.

Also, I discovered that food is fuel 100 per cent of the time and that what goes in the mouth has to be nutritionally worth it. And, if you are feeding yourself properly, you don't have to eat all the time—you can eat when you're hungry. What surprised me is that I can eat in a manner that feels natural to me. Eating nutrient-rich food just makes sense. This nutritional change was exciting—it felt like coming home. Also, I discovered that I can exercise reasonably and still keep my shape and weight.

The frustrating part was that the scale numbers didn't change fast enough for me. Cait said, "Wait for it—the body needs to trust to ADJUST." After eight weeks, suddenly the first 10 pounds dropped away. "Stick with it—change is slow." My body was holding back; it was not sure whether to trust that I was actually changing my eating philosophy. After 18 weeks, I lost 22 pounds, and best of all, I have more lean muscle mass and less fat.

My last thought is that it is true that when your food gets better, everything else gets better. Do your best to embrace this concept sooner rather than later.

CASE STUDY 9 (12 weeks)
The Twenty-Something: Avery's Story

Age: 23
Height 5'5"
Activity Level: high-intensity interval training three times per week, full-time child-care worker
Goal: To maintain a lean physique as I age and get my hormones and menstrual cycle back on track, along with my energy.

METRIC	START	12 WEEKS	TOTAL
Body Fat %	11.95	10.69	−1.26
Lean Pounds	116.23	117.88	+1.65
Fat Pounds	15.77	14.12	−1.65
Weight	132	132	0

Cait: Avery first came to me to workout. She wanted to stay lean and fit and was concerned that genetics would not be kind to her as she entered her thirties. Avery's first metric appointment showed her body fat at a lean 10.28 per cent. Her lean mass was 118.43 pounds; her body fat was 13.57 pounds. However, after a stressful career change and turning 25, Avery's answer was to eat less and work out more. Avery had a real fear of getting fat.

Her first metrics above are the ones I took one year after she started eating less and exercising more. Her body fat was only up a point or two, but her lean mass was down too! Her spark was gone, she was tired all the time, and she was moody. Most concerning was that Avery had developed amenorrhea—her menstrual cycle had stopped. She was living on about 600 to 700 calories per day and working out vigorously for an hour or more four to five days per week.

Feeling stuck, Avery decided to give NOURISH a try. Within three days of feeding her self enough nutrient-rich foods, Avery's energy returned, and she felt brighter. After two weeks of adding in more healthy fats, protein, and fibre, Avery could see a difference in her muscle tone. Here are her thoughts on NOURISH:

"I did NOURISH because I wanted to gain more knowledge and understanding about food and how it affects your body in both negative and positive ways. And how beneficial nutrient-rich food is to keep your body and mind in shape to handle the day-to-day things in life. I got results physically, mentally, and emotionally.

"Until I did my metrics in June, I didn't realize that I lost muscle and gained fat. However, over the year, I did notice a change in my body composition and the way my clothes fit. I was tired all the time and had lost definition in my muscle tone. After about four days into NOURISH, I started to notice the change in my stomach; I could finally start seeing the definition in my abs again.

"I started to realize that food is for fuel; we aren't eating for fun and to satisfy our taste buds. We are eating to survive and live a healthy life. Before NOURISH, I just ate what I was craving and when I was hungry. I never thought: "Why am I putting this into my body? How is it benefitting me?

"The lessons in NOURISH are something I will be able to use for the rest of my life and, someday, pass on to my children."

CASE STUDY 10 (12 weeks)
The Doctor: Rebecca's Story

Age: 53
Height: 5'6"
Activity Level: strength training two times per week, walking
Goal: To get rid of this middle-age spread!

METRIC	START	12 WEEKS	TOTAL
Body Fat %	21.47	16.78	−4.69
Lean Pounds	132.72	135.65	+2.93
Fat Pounds	36.28	28.93	−7.35
Weight	169	163	−6

My husband calls me the diet queen. He just rolls his eyes when I am reading yet another book on nutrition or trying another diet. I was fed up—literally—with diets and eating plans. I had reasonable success when I was young with popular diet programs. Unfortunately, I always seemed to lose a lot of weight and then gain it back over time. It has become harder over the years to lose weight. My monster cravings always seem to lurk just under the surface. Diet fatigue had set in, and I did not have much willpower when I started NOURISH. I was desperate to look and feel better. I was fearful of gaining more weight as I aged.

There are a number of things I like about this way of eating (I am refusing to call it a diet) and a number of things that really surprised me. First, I love being able to eat full fat. Now, we have one kind of milk in the fridge, instead of "his and hers." Also, I love being able to eat more protein. I always found that I felt better and was less hungry when I ate protein with every meal. I was shocked by my sugar intake. These were supposedly "good" sugars I was eating. No wonder I gained weight just looking at a small piece of chocolate! It always surprised me that a small indulgence, infrequently, could pack on a pound immediately. But, through TAAP, I learned that if you are scarfing down tons of sugar without realizing it, that little extra just tips the boat, doesn't it?

Carbohydrates: I thought I was doing well. Once again—NOT! But, it was easy to sort out. How? By eating more fat and cutting back on my sugar. Even the honey I loved so much in my tea had to go.

Within one week on NOURISH, I had no cravings. Within two weeks I was not looking for ways to "cheat." My constant hunger and cravings were gone. I think of this as mindful, preventative nutrition: feeding my body what it needs when it needs it. Keeping things from it that are harmful or unhealthy in the long term is not a hardship anymore—it has become a joy. NOURISH takes effort, but nothing worthwhile comes without effort. On those days when the mindful, preventative part feels too much for me, I just remember how I struggled to lose weight and about all the time I wasted in the past—and will waste again if I do not stick with this.

CASE STUDY 11 (12 weeks)
The Hunter: Bill's Story
Age: 59
Height: 5'9"
Activity Level: retired, golfer, walker
Goal: To avoid going on medication for high cholesterol, to increase my energy, and to improve sleep.

METRIC	START	12 WEEKS	TOTAL
Body Fat %	20.84	13.66	−7.18
Lean Pounds	163.87	175.27	+11.4
Fat Pounds	43.13	27.73	−15.4
Weight	207	203	−4

Cait: Bill came to me at his wife's request. Bill was 58 years old, retired, and his doctor wanted to put him on cholesterol medication. Golfing, walking his dogs every day, and eating healthy food was just not cutting it. His wife was frustrated because Bill did, in fact, eat well by today's mainstream standards:

little to no fat
plenty of whole grains
limited red meat (even though Bill is a hunter)
green tea
little to no alcohol

But, Bill had little-to-no energy, skin issues, lacked muscle tone, and his sleep was not restful. Bill also had a muffin top he could not seem to get rid of. He was feeling discouraged about the future because of his health.

Within two weeks of the program, Bill sent me this note:

"A quick update note...All is well. The best thing has been the blood-sugar fix. No more problems with my blood sugar crashing while walking the dog in the morning. I used to make sure I ate a large brunch before our hour-long hike but not anymore. And, the same thing is true with playing morning golf. Now, because I ate well the day before, I'm satisfied and full of energy the next morning. Still got a baby bump, but muffin top is dwindling."

CASE STUDY 12 (12 weeks)

The Professional: Jessica's Story

Age: 50
Height: 5'4"
Activity Level: high-intensity interval training three times per week, golf
Goal: Grow older gracefully and continue to enjoy playing golf!

METRIC	START	12 WEEKS	TOTAL
Body Fat %	23.94	12.07	−11.87
Lean Pounds	120.18	131.02	+10.84
Fat Pounds	37.82	17.98	−19.84
Weight	158	149	−9

I signed up for NOURISH because I felt fat (again), even though it was only a few pounds. I need accountability and a goal to work towards. My success with NOURISH comes down to a question Cait asked me at my metrics appointment: What would motivate me to become accountable to myself?

In the past five years, I had already made significant changes that were motivated by my quest for a healthier lifestyle. For NOURISH, instead of my typical "healthy lifestyle" answer, I was honest and shared that my motivation was to look good. I like seeing my muscles and feeling strong.

Now that I had my motivation, I was into the program a hundred per cent. I was eating new foods, thinking about healthy fats, decreasing my sugar intake, eliminating aspartame, TRACKing my food and water—and I saw results. The muffin top was disappearing, my biceps reappeared, I was starting to see my abs. And, I had no more headaches from the diet-pop habit or overloading on sugar. What tips would I give someone just starting out? Go cold turkey if you are quitting a bad habit—replace it with a new similar habit. At the beginning I was filling my pop bottles with water; I now have bottles of sparkling water to keep me from drinking regular pop. Keep TRACKing food and water—don't stop!

As I finished the program, I realize that the motivation for being accountable to myself will change as life progresses, and that's okay. The tools and lessons that I have learned from NOURISH are the foundation that will see me through those changes.

CASE STUDY 13 (12 weeks)
The Recovering Alcoholic: Dinah's Story

Age: 35
Height: 5'6"
Activity Level: yoga instructor, high-intensity interval training two times per week
Goal: I quit alcohol after almost dying. My next conquest was sugar. I came for the dress that I had to fit into for my sister's wedding but, I stayed for my well-being.

METRIC	START	12 WEEKS	TOTAL
Body Fat %	11.72	7.30	–4.42
Lean Pounds	135.96	138.13	+2.17
Fat Pounds	18.04	10.87	–7.17
Weight	154	149	–5

I came to Cait for vanity reasons—I wanted to look good in a dress. But, because of my years of seriously abusing alcohol, my internal organs were very damaged. I never felt well, I didn't have a lot of energy, my belly was always swollen, and I didn't feel good in my body overall.

Cait has a great line, "What got you here won't keep you here." When I first heard that, I realized that I came for a dress but stayed for my health. After living with liver disease for four years, I was sick and exhausted all the time. After doing NOURISH—and continuing to NOURISH my body properly for about a year—I have never been healthier in my whole life. NOURISH was an absolute life changer for me!

I first heard of Cait through a friend. I was looking for someone who could kick my ass back into shape and fit into a bridesmaid dress that I had already purchased. However, when I first began NOURISH, I realized what I had done was call Cait for help to quit sugar. As a recovering addict, I had come to physically depend on sugar the way my body used to depend on vodka. I found out in the first few weeks of taking all refined sugar out of my diet that my withdrawal symptoms from sugar were so similar to my alcohol withdrawal symptoms, it was scary.

The first thing I did was start TRACKing everything I ate. I learned that I wasn't eating enough, and what I was eating was crap. As a result of years of severely abusing alcohol, my digestive system was badly damaged. With NOURISH and because of TAAP, I was able to cope with the detox that came with quitting sugar cold turkey.

The longer I TAAP with my nutrition, the more and more I learn about myself. Since I've been out of rehab (three years), I've been working with a therapist and participating in activities that spark self-study and growth. I didn't ever think that nutrition would be one of them. One day, in a private session with Cait, she asked if I knew what diastasis recti was. It's something that happens to some women during pregnancy when the rectus abdominis muscles split. Only mine didn't happen during pregnancy, mine happened during the time I was in the hospital with severe liver and kidney failure, when my belly filled with fluid and I looked about 18 months pregnant. Cait taught me the correct way to engage my core while working out to heal my damaged abdominal muscles, and the correct way starts with the deep pelvic floor. This lesson led me to some more self-discovery: I realized that my disconnection with my sexual organs led from years of shame following being molested in my childhood and being raped in my teens. This realization has been a huge step for me. NOURISH gave me tools to heal my body, not only on the outside but my insides, too.

I'm in awe of my body and grateful every day for what it's capable of. The only tip that I would give to someone starting out would be to do the work required in NOURISH and TAAP. NOURISH was what I needed to get my whole self-healthy.

CASE STUDY 14 (12 weeks)
The Over-Exerciser: Tyson's Story
Age: 45
Height: 5'9"
Activity Level: High intensity interval training, three times per week, two distance runs and one yoga class
Goal: To manage stress and increase focus.

METRIC	START	12 WEEKS	TOTAL
Body Fat %	5.26	6.27	+1.01
Lean Pounds	137.37	139.65	+2.28
Fat Pounds	7.63	9.35	+1.72
Weight	145	149	+4

I solicited Cait's help with nutrition because, although I am fit and lean, I was interested in maintaining my health as I approach age 50.

The first thing I noticed TRACKing my food on the NOURISH program was how little calories I was consuming daily. Also, I was eating too little protein and consuming a lot of natural sugars in the form of fruit and higher sugar vegetables. Both of these habits made my appetite insatiable; I was always hungry.

Now, if I have an apple for a mid-morning snack, I make sure to have it with cheese. I cut back on the amount of berries I was eating to halve the sugar. I added other sources of healthy fats with fibre like chia and flax. Although my digestion has always been regular, I learned that eating enough fibre in my diet helps my guts in many ways including managing my monkey mind.

Just over six weeks into the program, my mind was more focused, and my sugar cravings were gone. My goal now is to continue to build more lean muscle.

An important point is this: I could not have known what was causing my constant state of hunger unless I TRACKed. Then, as NOURISH teaches, I ASSESSed and ADJUSTed my diet. You can make TAAP difficult or you can just embrace the process and do the work. I am eager to see what happens in the next few months.

CASE STUDY 15 (12 weeks)
The Teacher: Bethany's Story
Age: 41
Height: 5'4"
Activity Level: one strength training class and one Pilates class per week
Goal: Set a great example of healthy living for my two daughters and feel comfortable in my skin!

METRIC	START	12 WEEKS	TOTAL
Body Fat %	28.92	18.98	−9.94
Lean Pounds	110.89	118.29	+7.4
Fat Pounds	45.11	27.71	−17.4
Weight	156	146	−10

I have been on a roller coaster with weight my whole life. I was the queen of [popular diets], especially after each of my three children. I will admit the weight always came off but it eventually found its way back on. What I have learned through NOURISH is that my health cannot be determined by a number on a scale.

When my husband left me, I could not keep any food down at all. My insides were so torn up and my emotions were in such a jumble that the physical act of eating made me feel sick. Food would literally become lodged and I would have to force it up. This led me to be somewhat afraid to eat. This was something I never felt before, as I am a junk-food junkie, especially for salty snacks like chips and crispy French fries.

My weight dropped to an all-time low. Many people told me how "fabulous" I looked. But I felt like absolute crap on the inside, with no energy or drive.

Fast forward to today. Am I my ideal weight? No, I am not. I wouldn't even say that I am completely satisfied with my body and my eating habits. But, what I do know is that the knowledge I learned in NOURISH has helped me to understand that food in proper portions and combinations specifically for me can make me a powerhouse!

I have learned to forgive myself when I stray from the nutrition path, and to get back on the wagon as soon as possible and TAAP! I understand that there are foods (many that were staples on other diets I had tried) that contain absolutely no nutrition. And, if a food has no nutritional value, why put it in my mouth?

Through NOURISH, I am armed with the tools to help my two daughters make sensible food choices that make them feel strong and powerful. They understand that even "healthy" foods must be consumed in moderation and that excess sugar makes them feel rotten. My nine-year-old daughter is experiencing some health issues around anxiety. Cait and I discussed her food, and I was given suggestions that I never would have even considered! She had me TRACK if certain foods could be contributing to my child's anxiety. We've made some easy changes that have already started to make a difference.

So, am I the exact size I want to be right now? No! I have work to do. At 41 years old, it is a slower process than it used to be. NOURISH taught me to be patient and listen to my body. The best "meeting" I can go to: a good old-fashioned "check-in" with me. TRACKing my food helps me to ASSESS and then to ADJUST—to be accountable. That is real PROGRESS!

CASE STUDY 16 (12 weeks)
The Artist: Trina's Story
Age: 43
Height: 5'4"
Activity Level: light strength training, twice per week
Goal: Improve my monkey mind to help me focus on my passions and have more energy to do so!

METRIC	START	12 WEEKS	TOTAL
Body Fat %	29.84	23.06	−6.78
Lean Pounds	141.09	148.49	+7.4
Fat Pounds	59.91	44.51	−15.4
Weight	201	193	−8

My motivation for participating in NOURISH was to finally take charge of my poor eating habits. Since I was quite young, food was a comfort when I felt like something (love, affection, acceptance) was missing from my life. Food filled the void. As I got older and my excessive emotional eating led to an inevitable weight gain, that was useful to me as a kind of protection against unwanted attention from men. (I was sexually abused multiple times when I was young.)

The beauty of this program was that it wasn't offered as a means to lose weight. I have successfully lost weight (and regained it all, plus some) many times on diets geared solely toward dropping excess pounds. This program was my opportunity to finally understand how to best fuel my body in a way that would ultimately brighten and lighten my mind as well as my body. NOURISH did just that!

There was no mystery behind NOURISH. The lessons were straightforward and made a lot of sense. I was most struck by the fact that I wasn't following a generic diet plan. I was finally wrapping my head around my own nutritional tipping points and, at long last, given the knowledge and confidence to make changes that would better serve me through TAAPing.

The most difficult aspect of the program was the discipline required to diligently (and honestly) TRACK and ASSESS my food intake and the effects those foods had on my overall well-being. To be brutally honest, overcoming my self-sabotaging ways is still very much a work in progress.

The fact remains, as NOURISH teaches: once you learn something, you cannot unlearn it. I feel incredibly fortunate to have a firm grasp on how to best care for myself nutritionally, and that knowledge is empowering. I truly wish that everyone could have access to this program and be given the chance to ditch all of those old diet myths that have been working against them. Knowledge is power, and NOURISH sets you up for success!

CASE STUDY 17 (12 Weeks)
The Librarian: Judith's Story
Age: 52
Height: 5'2"
Activity Level: one Pilates class, one TRX strength training class, one yoga class
Goal: Stop dieting; start living!

METRIC	START	12 WEEKS	TOTAL
Body Fat %	30.95	27.43	−3.52
Lean Pounds	153.99	158.21	+4.22
Fat Pounds	69.01	59.79	−9.22
Weight	223	218	−5

I am a person who has always been on the heavier side of life. I use to say it was my "big bones" or family upbringing (always clean your plate) but I never admitted to my eating habits, until it was too late.

At 47 I was told I had Type 2 diabetes and I needed to change the way I ate. I also had high blood pressure, borderline high cholesterol, and a family history of heart attacks and strokes. I knew something had to change. I took the drastic step of gastric bypass surgery and thought,"I have fixed it now."

I was wrong.

Gastric bypass was just the first step. But, I needed to make sure that I didn't fall back into old habits. I needed to change the way I ate. I decided I would buy diet cereals, fruits, veggies, whole grains, diet granola bars, zero percent fat dairy and diet drinks as well as doing exercise and all would be fine, right?

Wrong. I needed to find foods that were good for me and understand what I'm eating and why the diet foods weren't helping me lose more weight. I needed to find out why I was tired, felt weak and had no energy.

I started exercise classes with Cait and heard everyone talk about NOURISH. Would it work for me? Dieting was not giving me the answer that I wanted.

The first thing that I learnt in NOURISH was that all my diet foods were lacking much of the nutrition I needed to power my system. I was exercising, and dieting but I wasn't feeding my body with food that would help sustain me. In other words, I was starving myself nutritionally. I needed to have foods that would be low in sugars, because of the diabetes, and give me the energy that I needed to keep me going.

The NOURISH lessons taught me that I need whole foods, with healthy fats, and I needed to balance what I ate for me personally. I needed to find my nutritional tipping points for protein, carbs, fats, sugars, etc. The joy of the lessons and the TRACKing was that I have this information to fall back on if I get derailed at any time. It is important to know what I am eating and why certain food is good for my body. Learning that I could eat whole foods again was so freeing! I no longer had to buy margarine, or low fat sour cream, diet yogurt or skim milk. My foods had flavour again and I enjoyed my meals.

It was tough unlearning all that I thought I knew was good. I am still trying to figure out how to make the changes I need as well as finding a way to get the calories I need into my meals so that I am not tired all the time or "starving" my body. I also drink a lot more water than I ever did. I didn't realize that the amount of water I drank each day would also affect my sleep and my digestion.

I still have slips, and I still have treats but I know that I am healthier for following the tools that I was given in NOURISH. I am building my muscle, and the fat is coming off. It is a slower process and it is sometimes confusing because I need to realize that I am adding muscle to my body as well as losing the fat that I want to. I need to stay off the scale and focus on TAAP and how I am feeling. I understand the wish to see the quick results but it is more important that I do it the right way and the healthy way. A diet will get you to the goal line but that is not good if you aren't eating healthfully and NOURISHing your body.

My goal for a healthier body is coming true because I have taken the path to a better way of eating. It is easy to maintain because the foods I eat are natural, healthy and regular items in my grocery store. I'm so glad I was able to take this course and learn how to NOURISH my body.

CASE STUDY 18 (12 Weeks)
The Photographer: Evangeline

Age: 43

Height: 5'4"

Activity Level: two, high intensity interval-training classes, one TRX strength class per week

Goal: Fat loss and to start seeing results for all my hard work!

METRIC	START	12 WEEKS	TOTAL
Body Fat %	37.78	32.25	−5.53
Lean Pounds	166.13	180.21	+14.08
Fat Pounds	100.87	85.79	−15.08
Weight	267	266	−1

I started to gain weight in my teen years once I got a driver's license. Before I drove a car, if I wanted to meet up with my friends, I had to walk or ride my bike. A round trip from home to where all the neighbourhood kids hung out was about four kilometres. I thought nothing of doing these treks three or four times a day. Once I could drive, my activity greatly decreased. I finished high school, took a two-year college program, and found a job in my field—a desk job where I sat for eight hours a day. Twenty-four years later, I am still at that job, sitting for eight hours a day. Having finished school, secured a good job, I married my high school sweetheart at 20. I had my first child at 22, and my second child at 26. I had it all and life was busy.

Although I had many activities that kept me active, such as gardening, home renovations, and running after two babies, they weren't enough. I was sitting at a desk for eight hours a day and eating a ton of sugar and other junk food to give me a rush and keep me going. I had every excuse in the book about why I couldn't exercise more, and although I had read a ton of information about "healthy" eating, I still had no idea what was healthy. The days and years rolled by and the pounds packed on. I'd try diet after diet, lose a few pounds, get discouraged, and gain back more weight than I had lost.

A year and a half ago, I decided enough was enough. I was 296 pounds, anxious, sad, and defeated. I did not feel like doing anything. My mother has terrible health issues, the majority of which are weight and lifestyle related. Her quality of life is so poor, and I felt as though I was looking in the mirror at [my] future unless I started to do something about it immediately.

I joined some exercise classes and started to eat in a way I felt was healthy. I used apps on my phone and plugged in all the numbers the app was looking for, and decided that a weight loss of two pounds per week was what I wanted. I lost about 30 pounds over a five-month period and I was thrilled. I joined a boot camp and also started taking various classes at Custom Fit. I had my metrics done as a starting point for my new-found exercise regime. I was working out three or four days per week. I was eating healthfully and exercising and logging my food.

I didn't lose a pound for seven months.

I had my metrics done again and discovered I had lost muscle. How was that possible when I was working out so much? Cait suggested that perhaps I was starving myself.

How could I be? I was eating 1,600-1,700 calories per day. It seemed like a high number, and the app said that was right for me if I wanted to lose weight. It didn't seem possible that I should eat more food to lose weight. It went against everything I thought I knew about weight loss. Something had to give!

Let me explain that over my year and a bit of working out and eating in a way that I thought was healthy, I felt a little less anxious and defeated, but I still did not feel great. My mind was over-active, my stress level was through the roof, and I often felt hungry, which inevitably led to frequent binges. I had somewhat let go of the idea that the number on the scale was the true victory, and started to embrace the idea of judging health by other factors, such as how my clothes fit or how I felt.

At one of my classes, Cait spoke about taking her NOURISH nutrition coaching course. A light bulb clicked on as though this may be my missing link. I had begun to establish a good routine for exercise and eating healthy, but there had to be something missing since I wasn't seeing the desired results. I signed up for NOURISH and it was truly the best thing I have ever done for myself.

I learned many things: I was starving myself; what nutrients my body needs and how much it needs; how essential fat is to my diet, and the difference between healthy fats and unhealthy fats; small changes lead to huge results; how much sugar is hidden everywhere in foods that have been marketed to us as "healthy"; that if NOURISH was going to work, I had to stop playing the victim and take control and plan ahead for times I knew I would have limited food choices; to bulk cook for the week; to prep my breakfast, lunch and snacks the night before and TRACK everything so I could ASSESS and ADJUST where necessary before I had eaten the food and it was too late.

At first, I felt like I was eating so much food that I couldn't possibly eat any more. I learned to add extra, nutritious foods to other foods, such as coconut oil, cacao nibs, hemp hearts, ground flaxseed to reach my daily nutritional requirements. I felt fabulous! I was getting compliments on my appearance, my skin felt soft, my complexion glowed, my eyes were bright, I had energy, my anxiousness was significantly reduced. I learned very quickly that if I had an "off-day," I felt horrible—sluggish, anxious, tired, which inevitably was accompanied by a headache.

What I learned, I cannot un-learn. I have gained knowledge that will serve me for the rest of my life. My body and mind are happy, and I will carry this knowledge with me through life. I feel as though I have finally achieved true health.

Knowledge is power!

CASE STUDY 19 (six months)

The Food-Phobic College Student: Vincent's Story

Age: 19
Height: 5'10"
Activity Level: non-exerciser
Goal: To overcome my phobia of food and to be kinder to my body.

METRIC	START	6 MONTHS	TOTAL
Body Fat %	13.69	6.85	−6.84
Lean Pounds	160.53	164.88	+4.35
Fat Pounds	25.47	12.12	−13.35
Weight	186	177	−9

Cait: Because of his school schedule, I checked in with Vincent at the six-month point, and he had dropped another three per cent body fat, added two more pounds of muscle, and lost another four pounds of fat. He looked healthy and brighter and was well on his way to overcoming his food-phobia issues. This is his story:

For most of my life, I have had an unhealthy relationship with food. For as long as I can remember, I have overeaten and rarely thought about the quality of the food that I was putting into my body. I knew a lot about nutrition, but rarely practiced it. However, within the last year, my eating habits changed drastically. I developed a severe anxiety disorder, which completely shifted my eating habits. I was diagnosed with Post Traumatic Stress Disorder (PTSD), and due to the nature of the trauma I experienced, I developed a phobic eating disorder. I had serious delusions about food and felt that eating posed a danger. It very quickly became easier to eat nothing than to deal with the inevitable panic that eating caused me.

Of course, depriving myself of nutrition only exacerbated the symptoms of my mental illness. I had serious blood sugar-regulation issues, completely lost my appetite, felt faint and would even black out when standing. My fasting only furthered my loss of contact with reality. Though weight loss was the last thing on my mind, I lost about 80 pounds in less than five months. When I did feel comfortable enough to eat, I lived off of sports drinks and simple carbohydrates—anything that would boost my blood sugar just enough to make me feel "normal"—only for me to feel as low as ever a couple of hours later.

When I began NOURISH, I saw huge changes from even the smallest steps. As I began to incorporate more brain-healthy fats into my diet, I found myself thinking more rationally, which reassured and inspired me to become more comfortable with food in general. As I ate more protein and cut out sugars, I found that I had much more physical energy and that my blood sugar began to regulate itself—no more faintness! Following NOURISH and TAAP, my relationship with food became consistently healthier, and so did my mental state.

I consider my change in diet to be the most important aspect of my rehabilitation (my psychiatrist was blown away that I had come so far and as quickly as I had using only therapy and nutrition and no drugs)! And though I never would have guessed that under eating would have been the catalyst for a drastically improved relationship with food, what I ended up learning from my experience and NOURISH is a gift that will benefit me for the rest of my life.

CASE STUDY 20 (two-years)
The Engineer: Jonathon's Story

Age: 56
Height: 5'10"
Activity Level: high-intensity interval training twice per week and yoga once per week
Goal: Improve my blood chemistry and keep up with my wife and daughter!

METRIC	2012	2014	TOTAL
Body Fat %	5.33	7.61	+2.28
Lean Pounds	148.64	158.91	+10.27
Fat Pounds	8.36	13.09	−4.73
Weight	157	172	+15

In the early summer of 2011, I considered myself to be active and in good health for my age. I was eating along government guidelines—lots of grains and veggies, not too much meat, hold the fat. I was 53 years old, 5' 10" tall and 185 pounds, with a 36" waist.

I compared my blood results with the Mayo Clinic targets: total cholesterol target was less than 5.2; I was 6.49. HDL (good cholesterol) target was greater than 1.6; I was 1.26. LDL (bad cholesterol) target was 2.6–3.3; I was 4.24. Triglyceride (blood sugar) target was less than 1.7; I was 2.17.

My question was, if I was following the government food guidelines, why was I outside the Mayo Clinic guidelines? I felt okay and my doctor didn't think any countermeasures were required at the time. But one thing that I couldn't understand was why I was so tired weekday afternoons. I literally fell asleep at my desk. I seriously considered buying a couch for my office so I could take a nap. I typically got up very early and kept busy all day, so I figured it must be due to that, plus my workload.

Was I wrong.

My story actually starts later that summer in 2011, with my wife and daughter. They joined Cait's cross-training classes at Custom Fit. All of a sudden, they were eating differently and doing all sorts of what I considered weird exercises. They were consuming fat and protein with limited amounts of good carbohydrates. They introduced new foods that I'd never even heard of, like chia seeds. I can vividly remember giving my wife the gears for eating so much cheese! Cheese contains a lot of fat, and that amount of fat wasn't recommended by government food guidelines.

In the winter of 2011, we travelled down south with the kids. I ran out of reading material, so I borrowed a book my wife had purchased as part of a wheat-free challenge she was participating in, under the guidance of Cait. The book was all about present-day GMO (genetically modified) wheat and how it is different from ancient wheat. I learned that today's finely ground, processed wheat was a simple sugar, very easily digested, quickly introduced into the blood stream, could spike your blood sugar, and was used in a staggering number of today's fast foods. I also learned that the gluten in wheat is an inflammatory and that it is not good for the brain or body. The pancreas secretes Insulin to reduce blood sugar. High blood sugar, over time, can lead to Insulin resistance and, eventually, type two diabetes. The book also talked about how blood sugar spikes causes Insulin spikes, resulting in low blood sugar, making you hungry for simple sugars again—basically a roller coaster of high/low blood sugar. Low blood sugar leaves you tired.

Was this what was happening to me weekday afternoons? I thought, what better way to prevent afternoon tiredness,

Insulin resistance, and possibly some aches and pains, than to try eliminating wheat from my diet. I was on my way.

I couldn't believe how many foods have wheat as an ingredient! We cleaned out our shelves; they were bare when we finished. Quite frankly, quitting products with wheat was overwhelming. What was there to eat if you eliminated all simple sugars? The cupboard was bare. The answer, of course, came with time and knowledge.

During the spring of 2012, we continued to eat wheat-free. We ate more protein and fats, plus good (complex) carbohydrates. I lost weight, I had more energy, and felt more alive. I noticed a couple other changes too. I used to get up in the morning and have to clear phlegm from my throat and nose. Since going wheat-free, my throat and nose were virtually clear. My wife's snoring dropped considerably as well.

The truth is, I got pretty lean when I first started eating like this—too lean, by Cait's standards. She asked me to adjust my diet a bit by consuming more healthy fats (like avocados) daily.

By fall of 2012 I was 157 pounds. I had my blood tested again. Total cholesterol target was less than 5.2; I was now 5.13 (-1.36). HDL (good cholesterol) target was greater than 1.6; I was 1.87 (+0.61). LDL (bad cholesterol) target was 2.6–3.3; I was 2.92 (-1.32). Triglyceride (blood sugar) target was less than 1.7; I was 0.74 (-1.43). Wow! My waist was now 32" (down from 36"). I ran the Terry Fox 10-kilometre run with my daughter. I wasn't tired in the middle of the afternoon anymore. I was feeling great!

In the winter of 2012, I was doing cross-training two times per week and doing yoga once per week. I was still eating wheat-free, a balance of protein and fats and complex carbohydrates. We stopped using rice, potato, and tapioca flours for bread and started to use only nut flours. I was eating mixed nuts as snacks. I was never hungry. I continued to feel great and looked forward to exercising.

And, all that high-intensity interval strength training combined with healthy eating had added lean muscle. How neat is that?

READER'S NOTES:

CASE STUDIES:
Tweens

Note: For the tween case studies, I asked the children to re-flect on their digestion, their sleep, their mood and their energy levels throughout the program. I kept the kids off the scale, and no metrics or photographs were taken.

CASE STUDY 21
Tween Girl: Louise's Story

Age: 11
Height: 5'3"
Activity Level: high-intensity interval training once per week, karate twice per week
Goal: To improve my confidence, mood and energy and get rid of the "hangries"!

One day last year, I went to the fridge to get a juice box. I opened the door, and there weren't any left. "Mom, where are the juice boxes?" I said.

"We won't be drinking juice anymore," she said.

At that moment, everything was different. No juice boxes for my lunch? No juice boxes as after-school snacks? When I finally got used to no more juice boxes I was fine without them. Then, suddenly, other things were gone too. "Hey, Mom, where is the bread? I was going to make a sandwich!" After about three months, everything sweet was gone, except ice cream on occasion. Then I started doing cross-train classes at Custom Fit one night a week.

A year later, things have changed a lot! My clothes fit better, and I eat healthier pretty much all the time, except for the occasional treat. I feel better about myself and how my skinny jeans fit. Before changing the way I eat, I wore a lot of baggy clothes because I felt like I was chubby. Now I like my clothes to fit me rather than hiding in big shirts over my skinny jeans. Also, I am a lot like my dad: when we get hungry we get the "hangries", and it's not fun for anyone—us included! I notice now that when I do eat a lot of junk food I don't feel as good. I get kind of whiny and tired, and I don't like that. I have more energy, and although I was always a good sleeper, I wake up less often with the "hangries". Eating healthy and watching out for sugar is just a way of life for me now. I don't miss the juice boxes at all!

CASE STUDY 22
Tween Boy: Benjamin's Story
Age: 12
Height: 5'4"
Activity Level: hockey, soccer, baseball
Goal: To be better at sports and be less anxious without medication.

I really love to play sports, and I play them year round. Even in between seasons, I play pickup games with my friends in my neighbourhood. So when I started to get headaches and stomach pains and didn't want to go to my practices, my mom got worried about me and took me to the doctor. The doctor told my mom that I needed medicine to make my brain "feel less anxious." My mom goes to Cait's classes, and it's a good thing, because Mom asked Cait if she thought eating better might help me. She said it might, and it turns out it did.

It's embarrassing to say this, but I wasn't going to the washroom every day. When Cait talked to me about food, we realized I was holding it until I got home; then I would forget about it and go to practice, get home, do homework, eat dinner, watch TV, and then go to bed. No trip to the washroom.

Also, I used to live on sports drinks and pop. I switched to just water, and my headaches started to go away. After giving it up, I had more energy in the morning and slept so much better at night. Mom makes sure I get enough protein every day now, too. I have really noticed a difference in my muscles. I am stronger during the off-ice training this year, and that makes me feel really good.

It's not like I never have treats—we have pizza every Friday night and Mom takes me for ice cream sometimes when we go to town. It's just that now I don't have pop, pizza, and ice cream all at the same time.

Mostly, I am so glad that I don't have to take medicine to make me feel calm.

READER'S NOTES:

PART VI
What Now?

CHAPTER TWENTY-THREE

The worst loneliness is to not be comfortable with yourself.
–Mark Twain

Be a Contender

I have an acquaintance that loses between 40 and 50 pounds every 18 to 24 months. Essentially, she starves herself thin. She will go food-free all day for a butter tart in the afternoon with the girls. Then she will eat tea and toast for dinner. She does this so she does not go over the daily permitted allotment of calories prescribed by the diet regime that has been her constant companion for much of her adult life. She's a believer, and hey, it does work. The fact that she is nutritionally bankrupt makes no difference to her. The fact that she does not exercise and takes a ton of medication doesn't matter either. Every 18 to 24 months, the number on the scale goes down. When she is lighter, that and that alone—that number on the scale—makes her a contender in life. The number on the scale is what allows her to shop where she wants to shop, on the size rack she thinks is respectable. She'll go on that trip of a lifetime, take her kids to the beach, allow someone to take her picture at functions, and have sex with her husband. The number on the scale gives her permission to enjoy the countless other nuggets in life that she denies herself when she is not the right number on the scale. Until, the number goes up on the scale again. Then, by her own admission, succumbing to the game that so many of us play but don't really know the rules to—she will no longer count. She will consider herself to be out of contention because of the number on the scale.

Until she is down…again.

I asked her the last time she lost weight, "What one thing will motivate you to keep going, to keep the weight off for good?"

Without hesitation she said, "Other people's compliments. It just feels so good to have people tell me how good I look now!"

I held my breath, bit the insides of my mouth, feigned a smile, and said, "Wow—it must feel really good when others acknowledge all of your hard work." (Because, make no mistake, starving one's self is *extremely* hard work.)

"It sure does," she beamed. "You know, just the other day, Suzie at the office pulled me aside and told me that she just couldn't get over just how great I looked. I was just so tickled."

Here's the thing: I happen to know for a fact that she loathes Suzie and has for 40 years. The notion that Suzie's approval was so important to this woman made me sad. And reflective…

I have a client who, several years ago, took the reins on her life. She did this with a massive change of attitude about what exactly she was responsible for in her own life like her food, her sleep, her fitness, her friends and, her overall lifestyle.

After shedding a ton of excess body fat through excellent nutrition, smart fitness, and calculated stress reduction, she proclaimed herself *a contender*. And today, years later, she still is. Life has changed with marriage and children and work schedules. When she falls off the wagon, she regroups swiftly and goes back to what works. Put plainly, she goes back to TAAP. Every time. She would be foolish not to! This is because once you learn what works for your body, you cannot un-learn it.

A Contender's Tried-and-True Systems:

Contenders cook in bulk. Every weekend, plan your week's meals, shop, wash and cut your veggies, and cook up your protein.

Contenders shop several times per week. If you're going to eat fresh, you have to buy fresh. This means one monthly trip to the big box store won't do it. The contender is not harried by this simple fact.

Contenders commit to an intelligent, purposeful fitness plan. Do both exercises you love (high intensity, cross-training) and ones that maybe you're not crazy about but know you need for stress reduction and balance (like yoga and Pilates). Or vice versa.

Contenders keep appointments with themselves. Put the oxygen mask on yourself first, by practicing self-care every day: eat well; hydrate; exercise; get enough sleep and, repeat daily.

Contenders keep food and exercise logs. With today's technology, this is a piece of cake. (TAAP). You have to TRACK in order to ASSESS, ADJUST, and make PROGRESS.

Contenders live. Never deny yourself birthday cake or good wine with great friends.

Falling Off of the Wagon

When you are a contender, your skin glows, your eyes are bright, and quite frankly, most people will never know when you are off track. But you will. And you will get off track—it's called *life*. When you do, just TRACK, ASSESS, ADJUST, and move on to PROGRESS. Contenders don't live in denial; they just get back on the wagon. As a contender, you have systems that work for you that you have honed throughout NOURISH with TAAP. Use TAAP when you fall off the wagon. As long as you are right with yourself, practice caring less about what others think. As a contender, do this, all of this, for yourself. This, and this alone, makes you a contender.

CHAPTER TWENTY-FOUR

I realize that I've been using my politeness as an excuse to indulge.
–Jessica, NOURISH client

Social Gatherings

Let's say you are headed to a party. During the day, drink your water, keep your carbs limited to low-sugar, higher-fibre vegetables and fruits: cucumbers, broccoli, cauliflower, greens, berries, and avocados (i.e. limit red peppers, carrots, or high-sugar fruits like apples or bananas). Before you head out, make sure you have consumed enough protein and fats throughout your day so you are well NOURISHed.

Once at the party, plan your food. This means that if you are at the buffet table snacking, stick to low-sugar, higher-fibre vegetables and cheeses. Lunch meats are full of nitrates, monosodium glutamate (MSG), and gluten—stay away from them at all costs. You can take a chance on shrimp and pray it is wild caught (you could ask if you feel comfortable).

When you sit down for the meal, if you want nutrient-dead bread, consider whether you want to eat cake later. Ask yourself if you really need both? How will you feel tomorrow? You may have to decide: bread now or cake later. Same goes for alcohol—don't drink sugary alcoholic beverages all night long. If you must drink, stick to vodka or tequila. Dry wine is okay as long you know how it affects you. And, keep drinking water throughout the evening!

Consider this: it's usually the first bite or sip of something that give us the most pleasure—not the 30th.

The most important piece of advice I can give you is to get right back into your routine the next morning. Do not let one night of over indulgence turn into a weekend bender. I see this with clients who turn a one week, all-you-can-eat cruise into a six month, self sabotage, junket! One night of sin won't make a difference that you cannot recover from within 24 to 36 hours. Multiple days, weeks, months or years of poor choices take a lot more work. Also, resist the urge to eat well all week and then binge all weekend. Why would you build a foundation for your house every Monday and then knock it down every Thursday afternoon for a three daylong happy hour?

CHAPTER TWENTY-FIVE

Bring the best of who you are.
–Linda Kelliher

What Brought You Here Can't Keep You Here

Here is a scenario for you…You do the NOURISH program. You TRACK, ASSESS, ADJUST…you make PROGRESS! You finish your halfway metrics; you complete your 12 weeks metrics. All of your PROGRESS is backed up by your data for your metrics, your photos, your target outfit and how you *feel*. The timeline of the NOURISH program plays out like this:

First you *feel* a difference.

Then you *see* a difference.

Then other people *feel* a difference in you.

Then, other people *see* a difference in you.

Other people notice that you are somehow "different." And, different on the NOURISH program is polite code for better! They are complimenting you.

You ARE "different!" You have been focusing on your self-care by establishing nutritional tipping points that serve you.

You finish the book. You are "free"…

You decide you'll "take a break as a bit of a reward." You deserve it, right? You worked hard! Maybe you made huge, sweeping changes to your diet; maybe you discovered how a series of small changes bring big results. Yay you! You've got this…

You stop TRACKing your food for a day or two which turns into a week, a month…six months. You revert back to old eating habits from week number one. Except:

You put chia seeds on your processed cereals.

You continue to eat avocado daily and you hit the drive thru for the mid-morning bagel.

You have a lunchmeat, nitrate laden, sub for lunch (no mayo) and you put coconut oil in your tea.

You eat full fat yogurt but add back the honey.

You keep your protein smoothie for breakfast and add back the banana and magoes because, darn it— *you like them!*

You have pasta for dinner but make sure to add olive oil.

You stop drinking your daily water minimum. Hey, you're not that thirsty and did the water really make that much of a difference?

For convenience, you switch back to store bought dressings and you pick up the "lite" version out of habit and because your spouse in not on board with the teachings of NOURISH.

You revert back to the Sunday morning ritual of pancakes for the kids. Come on! They're kids...

Weekly pizza night returns...

Or, maybe you will go back to what was unintentionally starving yourself to now *intentionally* starving yourself because, once you know you cannot un-know.

Soak on that one for a moment...

Whatever you do, choose one scenario or the other. Do what worked for you while on NOURISH, or choose to go back to your old ways. Do one or the other. My advice is to go back and re-read your reasons for wanting to do the NOURISH program. Revisit your first couple of food logs. Think about how you feel now compared to when you started. Look at your PROGRESS!

I mentioned in the introduction that the 80/20 rule is a myth. You can't "live well all week" and then "go hog wild" every weekend and start fresh on Monday mornings. You will only get away with this for so long and then the body will fight back. For you this might mean:

- having digestive issues

- experiencing headaches
- suffering from joint pain
- storing excess body fat
- succumbing to moodiness
- enduring night sweats
- serious disappointment in yourself for knowing better...

It's all about choices. "Have to" or "Choose to." It's up to you.

Here are some final thoughts from NOURISH clients:

Understanding the why for me was easy. Implementing change without making excuses is the challenge. I used food in emotional or stressful situations, either eating junk or skipping meals. Recognize that you are responsible for bad choices, not those around you.

–Jessica, NOURISH client

Like nutrition, the body is always evolving and changing, and so you must too, if progress is to be maintained and improved upon. My next goal is to get my family on board with eating properly and am excited to see the changes or "aha" moments it brings for them.

–Dinah, NOURISH client

Today, at age 57, I have five grandchildren, and I embrace and enjoy life with strength and a relaxed, calm energy. Fuelling my body with the right food is my highest priority. Buying, planning, and preparing meals and snacks, always thinking ahead for my work day, weekend day trips, vacations, or last-minute changes in plans; this ready-for-anything strategy has become an integral part of who I am.

–Bonnie, NOURISH client

If people want to make changes in their lives—to feel better, look better, sleep better—then they have to make the commitment to record their food. It is also harder to eat junk if you have to record it—even if you are the only one who sees it.

–Meghan, NOURISH client

Question: Do I still have to TAAP?
Answer: That is totally up to you.

In my experience, it is easy to slide back into old patterns. Even if you have cut back on sugar and trips to fast-food restaurants, how do you know if you are drinking enough water every day or if you are getting enough fibre? Are you consuming too much protein? Are you eating enough nutrient-rich calories daily? How much healthy fats are you eating a day? You simply cannot know unless you TRACK.

I had an eye-opener when I started weighing my avocados.

When I TRACKed, for convenience, I typed in one avocado. But, 100 grams of avocado has 6.7 grams of fibre and one, whole Florida or California avocado has13.5 grams of fibre! That's a huge difference between the one avocado and the measured avocado. Can you see how, without measuring, if I had a small avocado compared to a large avocado (156 grams) my nutrients for my whole day would change? And, not just fibre but fats, calories, and carbs too!

Here are some thoughts from Justine after she quit tracking over the holidays:

> "In my wisdom, I thought it would be smart to stop tracking, which obviously was the worst mistake I could make. My mood suffered and too much sugar made for some pretty horrible digestion. The good news is I'm getting it together and know exactly what I need to do to get back on TAAPing and making smarter decisions."

Here is an example of proactive planning from Bonnie:

> "When we're away for the weekend, vacation, or even for the day, we always bring nuts, dark chocolate, and a shaker bottle, along with protein powder and chia powder. (My husband doesn't like the clumpy texture

of chia seeds but finds the chia powder is okay). The protein mixed with chia truly does replace a meal when needed. And the shaker bottles are fantastic for water; the wide-mouth screw-off top lets you refill even from a water fountain at the airport."

Personally, I use TAAP more often than I do not. It keeps me on target with my goals that are to have a digestive system that functions in a reliable way and to sleep well and feel restored and refreshed every morning (and to wake before my alarm). I like to have a focused, clear mind and positive outlook and I enjoy energy that is manageable. This means high when I need it or calm when appropriate

Every time I stray from TAAP, I lose ground that I then have to make up. To me, this is lost time. However, when I do fall off the wagon and stop TRACKing my food, water, and exercise, the easiest way that I know to get back on the wagon is to TAAP. Some people only TAAP during the week and then take a break on the weekend. In my opinion, you have to be very dedicated to your food sources and prepared to make this work. Otherwise, you might be trying to live on the 80/20 system: eating well 80 per cent of the time and not eating well the other 20 per cent. This simply is not healthy in the long term. It is an example of yo-yoing. You might eat that way on holidays, but as soon as you return from the trip or Thanksgiving is over, the goal has to be to eat well 100 per cent of the time. And, as I hope you know by now, that does not mean you cannot have cake on your birthday! Yes, have the cake, but plan your nutrition around the extra carb and sugar intake that day and the day after. Also, make sure you get the good, nutrient-rich foods into you even if you are over your calories that day. Starving yourself to eat cake always backfires.

A note from Ed about falling off the wagon:

"I fell off the wagon twice early on in NOURISH (and I have again since), once with an injury and once with the arrival of our baby. You would not believe how fast I felt poorly again. But, I am back on

TRACK now. It really is pretty easy to correct things, to get back into TAAP. If you screw up, just start again!"

The problem is not that we fall off the wagon; it's that we lie under the wagon and wallow. Always remember that you are learning, not failing.

Some final advice from Ed:

"Do not fight the system or complain about it. Listen, learn, and grow with it. It is a life-changer.."

Good advice. Stay curious.

Notes

[1] Marcelle Pick, OB/GYN, "Psychological Symptoms of Adrenal Fatigue," https://www.womentowomen.com/adrenal-health-2/psychological-symptoms-of-adrenal-fatigue/. (Accessed August 10, 2015.)

[2] The American Academy of Orthopedic Surgeons, "Effects of Aging," Ortho Info. http://orthoinfo.aaos.org/topic.cfm?topic=A00191. (Accessed May 21, 2015.)

[3] Web MD, "Sarcopenia With Aging", http://www.webmd.com/healthy-aging/sarcopenia-with-aging. (Accessed May 21, 2015.)

[4] Anne Marie Helmenstine, Ph.D., "How Much of Your Body is Water?", http://chemistry.about.com/od/waterchemistry/f/How-Much-Of-Your-Body-Is-Water.htm. (Accessed May 25, 2015.)

[5] webmd.com, "The Truth About Fat," http://www.webmd.com/diet/features/the-truth-about-fat?page=2 (Accessed July 15, 2014.)

[6] Sally Tamarkan, "34 Proven Ways Water Makes You Awesome." http://greatist.com/health/health-benefits-water. (Accessed January 6, 2015.)

[7] Sophie C. Killer, Andrew K. Blannin , Asker E. Jeukendrup, "No Evidence of Dehydration with Moderate Daily Coffee Intake: A Counterbalanced Cross-Over Study in a Free-Living Population," PLOS ONE. Published: January 9, 2014. http://journals.plos.org/plosone/article?id=10.1371/journal.pone.0084154. (Accessed May 21, 2015.)

[8] Oxford Dictionaries, http://www.oxforddictionaries.com/definition/english/basal-metabolic-rate. (Accessed July 12, 2014)

[9] The Free Dictionary by Farlex http://www.thefreedictionary.com/catabolism. Accessed May 14, 2015.

[10] Source for TDEE: http://calorieline.com/tools/tdee

[11] Wikipedia., Harris–Benedict Equation. http://en.wikipedia.org/wiki/Harris%E2%80%93Benedict_equation. (Accessed May 14, 2015.)

[12] Institute of Medicine, "Dietary Reference Intakes for Energy, Carbohydrate, Fiber, Fat, Fatty Acids, Cholesterol, Protein, and Amino Acids," http://www.iom.edu/reports/2002/dietary-reference-intakes-for-energy-carbohydrate-fiber-fat-fatty-acids-cholesterol-protein-and-amino-acids.aspx, September 5, 2002. (Accessed July 12, 2014.)

[13] The Free Dictionary by Farlex. http://medical-dictionary.thefreedictionary.com/protein+turnover. (Accessed May 9, 2015.)

[14] Joseph Mercola, "Soy: This 'Miracle Health Food' Has Been Linked to Brain Damage and Breast Cancer," mercola.com, http://articles.mercola.com/sites/articles/archive/2010/09/18/soy-can-damage-your-health.aspx. (Accessed July 22, 2014.)

[15] Nina Teicholz, "The Questionable Link Between Saturated Fat and Heart Disease," The Wall Street Jorunal (online), May 6, 2014. (Accessed July 16, 2014) http://www.wsj.com/articles/SB10001424052702303678404579533760760481486

[16] Joseph Mercola. "Fat, Not Glucose, is the Preferred Fuel for Your Body." http://fitness.mercola.com/sites/fitness/archive/2012/08/10/fat-not-glucose.aspx, August 12, 2012. (Accessed August 20, 2014).

[17] Dr Ananya Mandal, "What are Hormones?" http://www.news-medical.net/health/What-are-Hormones.aspx. (Accessed May 20, 2015.)

[18] Joseph Mercola, "Coconut Oil vs. Vegetable Oils: What Oil Should You Be Cooking with, and Which Should You Avoid?" http://articles.mercola.com/sites/articles/archive/2003/10/15/cooking-oil.aspx. (Accessed August 15, 2014.)

[19] Food Choices and Coronary Heart Disease: A Population Based Cohort Study of Rural Swedish Men with 12 Years of Follow-up, October 12, 2009. http://www.mdpi.com/1660-4601/6/10/2626. (Accessed May 10, 2015.)

[20] Nora T. Gedgaudas, CNS, CNT *Primal Body, Primal Mind*, (Rochester, Vermont: Healing arts Press, 2011) p 113.

[21] Mayo Clinic Staff, "Trans fat is double trouble for your heart health." http://www.mayoclinic.org/diseases-conditions/high-blood-cholesterol/in-depth/trans-fat/art-20046114. (Accessed May 111, 2015.)

[22] Christian Nordqvist, "What are carbohydrates? What is glucose?" Medical News Today, http://www.medicalnewstoday.com/articles/161547.php (Accessed May 7, 2015.)

[23] Christine Wilcox, "Understanding Our Bodies: Insulin." http://nutritionwonderland.com/2010/05/understanding-our-bodies-insulin/. (Accessed August 24, 2014.)

[24] Mayo Clinic Staff Dietary fiber: Essential for a healthy diet http://www.mayoclinic.org/healthy-lifestyle/nutrition-and-healthy-eating/in-depth/fiber/art-20043983

[25] Joseph Mercola, "The Health Benefits of Fiber," November 25, 2013. http://articles.mercola.com/sites/articles/archive/2013/11/25/9-fiber-health-benefits.aspx. (Accessed August 1, 2014.)

²⁶ Elissa M. Howard-Barr, "Fibre." http://www.faqs.org/nutrition/Erg-Foo/Fiber.html. (Accessed May 22, 2014.)

²⁷ The American Heart Association, Circulation: Journal of the American Heart Association, August, 2009.

²⁸ Rada P1, Avena NM, Hoebel BG, "Daily bingeing on sugar repeatedly releases dopamine in the accumbens shell." National Institutes of Health: http://www.ncbi.nlm.nih.gov/pubmed/15987666. (Accessed May 12, 2015.)

²⁹Patrick J. Skerrett,"Is fructose bad for you?" Harvard Health Publications, http://www.health.harvard.edu/blog/is-fructose-bad-for-you-201104262425, April 26, 2011. (Accessed May 21, 2015.)

³⁰World Health Organization Sugars intake for adult and children. Guideline http://www.who.int/nutrition/publications/guidelines/sugars_intake/en/ http://www.who.int/mediacentre/factsheets/fs394/en/ Healthy Diet Fact Sheet May 2015.

³¹ http://www.cbsnews.com/news/world-health-organization-lowers-sugar-intake-recommendations/

³² Names for sugar list adapted from: CRISTIANO LIMA, "The 57 Names Of Sugar," http://www.prevention.com/food/healthy-eating-tips/57-names-sugar, October 15, 2013. Accessed November 13, 2014).

³³ George Dvorsky, "Why We Need To Sleep In Total Darkness," io9 We Come from the Future, http://io9.com/why-we-need-to-sleep-in-total-darkness-1497075228. January 8, 2014. (Accessed January 10, 2014.)

³⁴ American Psychological Association "Why sleep is Important and What Happens When you Don't Get Enough," http://www.apa.org/topics/sleep/why.aspx. (Accessed May 23, 2015.)

Acknowledgements

I had some crazy "who luck" on this project…

First, thank you to my husband Derek and daughter Lila for all of their patience and support. Thank you to my mom, Isla Awen, for instilling in me curiosity. Thanks to my dad, Tom Curley, for passing down his tenacity and drive. Thank you to my in-laws, Dave and Linda Lynch. Without them helping to care for our daughter, it would have been a challenge to complete this project!

Thanks to my Aunt FAB, Elizabeth Casey, for her efforts and grammar policing in the early editing of my first draft.

Lessons learned: Show gratitude to those you love; be grateful for where you came from.

Thanks to Carey Dinkel for encouraging me not to pull the plug on the whole thing in the summer of 2014 when we sat together at lunch and I confided that I didn't think it could be done. She disagreed…Thanks for being an early, patient reader as well.

Thanks to Jen Stewart for keeping Custom Fit humming along behind the scenes. I so appreciate Jen and what she does!

Thanks to Chef Cuddy, Stephanie Cudmore—she is a steady and loyal friend.

Thanks to Kirk Mechar for telling me I "had to write a book." He was right—I had to do this and I'm so glad that I did. Kirk edited draft after draft, all the way through, and is still speaking to me! He is the perfect combination of devil's advocate and cheerleader. Kirk always asks, "What's the solution?" and I am most grateful for that.

Thank you to my dearest friend in the world, Linda Kelliher. Thanks also to Tamara Jones, Jon Testa and Sarah Ostrofsky at Linda's company, Kelliher, Samets and Volk

(KSVC.COM). Tamara and Jon whipped out the graphics for the book in no time flat and Sarah helped bring the cover design to life.

Lessons learned: Surround yourself with great people and ask for help when you need it.

Thank you to all the Custom Fit Nutrition Coaching clients from fall of 2009 to right this moment. I learned so much from all of you!

Lesson learned (and lived): Do what you love. We should and I do.

In January of 2015, during our first week back to classes at Custom Fit, at the end of each class, our clients shared their goals for the New Year. At one of the last classes of the week, after listening to everyone else's goals and recording each of them for them, scribbling as fast as I could, someone said, "Cait! What about you? What's your goal for 2015?"

"My goal is to find a publisher for my book," I said.

From saying that simple statement out loud, two very important things happened:

> Ann Oliphant sent me a note the next day about a friend of hers who "edits books for a living."
> Pam Vorkapic told me that her "boss owned a publishing company."

Thank you to Sarah Jacob and Shane Joseph of Blue Denim Press for taking on this project and bringing a big dream to life!

The lesson I learned from this is to open the closet door on your goals and share them! You never know—as long as you do the work required—just how "who luck" will show up for you.

Lessons learned: Write your goals down and declare them. Truly.

And, finally (humour me because I'm wired this way), thank you to Betty the dog, my constant writing companion and loyal friend.

Lesson learned: There is nothing like a great dog.

About the Author

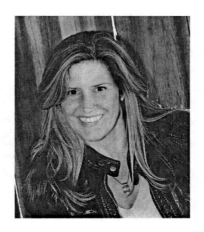

Since 2004, Cait Lynch has owned and operated Custom Fit Vitality where she coaches nutrition, fitness, and momentum. Having coached people both on the ground and on horseback for over twenty-five years, Cait's direct and passionate approach blends into everything she offers to the communities she serves. Seeing the light go on for clients is what makes Cait bounce out of bed every day. Cait lives with her husband and daughter on their horse farm in Ontario, Canada.

Visit Cait at: WWW.CAITLYNCH.COM
WWW.CUSTOMFITVITALITY.COM

Resources

Calories:

Total Daily Energy Expenditure (TDEE): You can check out this site:
http://www.myfitnesspal.com/topics/show/653038-how-to-calculate-your-tdee-made-simple
J. Arthur Harris and Francis G. Benedict, "A Biometric Study of Human Basal Metabolism."
http://www.ncbi.nlm.nih.gov/pmc/articles/PMC1091498/?tool=pubmed

More on harmful oils:

http://articles.mercola.com/sites/articles/archive/2003/10/15/cooking-oil.aspx

More on sugar:

Sugar: The Bitter Truth
http://www.youtube.com/watch?v=dBnniua6-oM

Fat Chance, Fructose 2.0
http://www.youtube.com/watch?v=ceFyF9px20Y

More on sleep:

Joseph Mercola, "How the Cycles of Light and Darkness Affect Your Health and Wellbeing," mercola.com, January 19, 2014.
http://articles.mercola.com/sites/articles/archive/2014/01/19/sleep-light-exposure.aspx

More on exercise:
http://bodyforlife.com/library/exercise/cardio

Lyme Disease:
Under Our Skin: A Documentary
http://www.underourskin.com
Canadian Lyme Disease Foundation:
http://canlyme.com/
http://www.lymemd.org
Dr. Richard Horowitz: http://www.cangetbetter.com (my Lyme doctor in 2000)

BOOKS
Why Can't I Get Better?: Solving the Mystery of Lyme & Chronic Disease, by Dr. Richard Horowitz
Deep Nutrition: Why Your Genes Need Traditional Food, by Catherine Shanahan and Luke Shanahan
Food Rules, by Catherine Shanahan
The Essentials of Sport and Exercise Nutrition, by John Berardi, PhD and Ryan Andrews, MS, MA, RD
Why We Get Fat, by Gary Taubes
The End of Overeating, by David A. Kessler, MD
The Paleo Solution, by Robb Wolf
The Primal Blueprint, by Mark Sisson
The Fat Switch, by Richard J. Johnson, MD
Clean, by Alejandro Junger, MD
Wheat Belly, by William Davis, MD
Grain Brain, by David Perlmutter, MD
The Paleo Diet, by Loren Cordain, PhD
Lights Out, by T. S. Wiley with Bent Formby, PhD
Women Food and God, by Geneen Roth
The China Study, by T. Colin Campbell, PhD and Thomas M. Campbell II PhD
The Omnivore's Dilemma, by Michael Pollan
Fat Chance, by Robert H. Lustig, MD, MSL
It Starts with Food, by Dallas and Melissa Hartwig

The Carbohydrate Addict's Diet, by Dr. Rachel F. Heller and Dr. Richard F. Heller
How to Eat, Move, and Be Healthy, by Paul Chek
Spark, by John J. Ratey, MD
The War on Art, by Steven Pressfield

Films:
Food Inc.
Fed Up
Hungry for Change

Websites:
Mercola.com
ChrisKesser.com
weightymatters.ca
wellnessmama.com
trimhealthymama.com
www.ericcressey.com

CPSIA information can be obtained at www.ICGtesting.com
Printed in the USA
LVOW10s2005220416

484938LV00013B/91/P

9 781927 882160